ARE POISONING YOUR PETS?

Nina Anderson
Howard Peiper

Illustrated by Richard Vail

Avery Publishing Group
Garden City Park, New York

The information, advice, and procedures contained in this book are based upon the research and the personal and professional experiences of the authors. They are not intended as a substitute for consulting with a veterinarian or other qualified healthcare provider. Because there is always some risk involved, the author and publisher are not responsible for any adverse effects or consequences resulting from the use of any of the suggestions, preparations, or methods described in this book. The publisher does not advocate the use of any particular diet or health program, but believes that the information presented in this book should be available to the public.

This text is as timely and accurate as its publisher and authors can make it. All listed addresses, phone numbers, and fees have been reviewed and updated during the production process. However, the data is subject to change. Refer to other current sources of information to verify textual material.

Cover design: William Gonzalez
Cover photo: Stock Imagery
Illustrator: Richard Vail
In-house editors: Helene Ciaravino and Jennifer Santo
Printer: Paragon Press, Honesdale, PA
Typesetter: William Gonzalez

Avery Publishing Group
120 Old Broadway
Garden City Park, NY 11040
1–800–548–5757

Library of Congress Cataloging-in-Publication Data

Anderson, Nina, 1948–
    Are you poisoning your pets? : a guidebook to how our lifestyles
    affect the health of our pets / by Nina Anderson and Howard Peiper ;
    illustrated by Richard Vail.
        p.   cm.
    Includes bibliographical references and index.
    ISBN 0–89529–829–5
    1. Veterinary toxicology.   2. Pets—Health   3. Household
    supplies—Toxicology.   I. Peiper, Howard.   II. Title
    SF757.5.A63   1998
    636.088í7—dc21   98–4712
                                                                  CIP

Printed in the United States of America

10 9 8 7 6 5 4 3 2 1

Table of Contents

*We dedicate this book to all of our animal friends
who trust us to give them not only our love,
but to choose the right food for them and to
provide a healthy place in which they can live.*

Acknowledgments

We acknowledge our spouses, who kept our animals off the computer and took care of them while we toiled away in research for endless hours. Also, to all the companies who appear in the Product Directory, we give you thanks for the much needed technical research that you provided and for your devotion to our furry and feathered friends.

Foreword

The commonplace, everyday products that we purchase for ourselves, our homes, and our animal companions often contain hidden dangers. Some of these substances can even be life-threatening. You are about to read a very informative, well-written book on a subject that, unfortunately, receives little attention—how these hazardous materials affect our pets.

The authors of this book have compiled an eye-opening, comprehensive summary of potentially toxic substances found in and around the home. The text begins with information on building and decorating materials, and continues with discussions on carbon monoxide, cleaning products, lead, dangerous plants, pesticides and flea treatments, and water contamination. It concludes on an optimistic note, offering valuable information on such subjects as diet, exercise, helpful remedies, and healthy air for our pets. Nina Anderson and Howard Peiper not only alert us to the threat of pet poisoning, but also offer us solutions.

At a time when chronic diseases such as cancer in animals are on the upswing and nearly in an epidemic state, *Are You Poisoning Your Pets?* investigates some possible underlying causes. The authors explore the problem at its roots and promote the prevention of avoidable sickness. Perhaps we should spend more time eliminating toxic materials from our homes and our environment, and then take special note of what happens to the incidence of degenerative illnesses in both animals and people.

—Robert S. Goldstein, V.M.D.
Holistic Veterinarian
Co-editor of *Health Animals*
Phillips Publishing of Potomac, Maryland

Introduction

Are you poisoning your pet with building and decorating materials, chemical cleaners, pesticides, and contaminated water? Is your home actually a *hazard zone* for your animal companion? This book discusses the possible dangers to which you unknowingly may be exposing your pet. In addition, because healthy animals have better luck at fending off toxic assaults than unhealthy ones, we include a chapter on strengthening your animal's immune system through proper nutrition and lifestyle. Finally, at the conclusion of this text, we provide a Product Directory, listing products that are conducive to a healthier pet and home.

In its agenda to promote good health and a safe environment, the media has exposed a great deal of information on the subject of indoor air pollution. For example, the *Journal of the American Medical Association* reports that the incidence of respiratory infection is 45 percent higher among occupants of new buildings than those of older ones. Modern energy-efficient construction methods are most likely the responsible agent; in their function to provide superior insulation, these methods prevent air from leaking into or out of the house. While the newer techniques save you a great deal of money in heating costs, they also result in a build-up of chemical fumes within the home. And as pets spend much of their time indoors, they may be developing serious health problems. We must not forget that our animals are closer to the contaminating source for more time than we are, and that they breathe in even higher concentrations of the toxins, considering the ratio of body weight to amount inhaled. If we are using materials that contain formaldehyde, plastics, synthetics, petroleum products, etc., all of which release harmful fumes into the indoor air, then we should be putting gas masks on our pets!

Older homes contain their own health hazards, primarily because paint manufactured before 1978 contains lead. This can cause severe problems, especially in puppies who may either chew painted wood or inhale lead dust. Regardless of when a home was built, the average house stocks potentially dangerous substances. Household cleaners can be extremely toxic to pets, as can common bug sprays and garden pesticides. Even certain potted plants and common tap water can negatively affect your pet's health.

Many books have been written about household dangers and their associated health implications for humans. The media has covered stories about toxic carpets and lead paint ingestion. Newspapers and magazines often report on the tragedies of carbon monoxide poisoning in the home. Numerous health articles about mold allergies are published during the start of the heating season. But almost no studies are done concerning the effects of construction materials, household products, and pollutants on the millions of family pets. Veterinarians are treating more and more cases of cancer in animals, as well as increased numbers of behavioral problems and poisonings. Cats, in particular, have difficulty eliminating toxic chemicals because their systems are inefficient at metabolizing foreign intruders. We must educate ourselves because the substance- and product-related illnesses from which our pets suffer are often preventable.

This book is intended to serve as a guide to preventing pet sickness. It teaches you how to provide a safe environment for your animal companion, how to be responsible in your use of household products, and economical ways to change consumer habits. Every home can have both modern luxuries *and* healthy pets, if precautions are taken.

Trouble-Shooting Table
Symptoms & Sources of Pet Poisoning

The following table lists a number of symptoms and identifies toxic sources that may be causing each of them. If your pet is experiencing any of these symptoms, turn to the appropriate chapters for more information and be sure to contact a veterinarian to further discuss and treat the animal's condition.

Symptoms	Possible Sources
Aimless running	Dogs: lead
Anorexia	Cats: pesticides and flea repellents; contaminated water
	Dogs: lead; pesticides and flea repellents; contaminated water
Anxiety	Birds: building and decorating materials; cleaning products
	Cats: building and decorating materials; cleaning products
	Dogs: building and decorating materials; cleaning products

Symptoms	Possible Sources
Asthma	Cats: cleaning products Dogs: cleaning products
Blindness	Dogs: lead
Breathing problems (*see also* increased respiratory rate; panting; respiratory stress and possibly failure; shallow breathing; shortness of breath; slow respiration)	Birds: building and decorating materials; carbon monoxide; cleaning products; pesticides and flea repellents Cats: building and decorating materials; carbon monoxide; cleaning products; pesticides and flea repellents; toxic plants Dogs: building and decorating materials; carbon monoxide; cleaning products; pesticides and flea repellents; toxic plants
Burns on the mouth and esophagus	Birds: cleaning products Cats: cleaning products Dogs: cleaning products
Cancer	Birds: building and decorating materials; contaminated water Cats: building and decorating materials; pesticides and flea repellents; contaminated water Dogs: building and decorating materials; pesticides and flea repellents; contaminated water
Cardiac arrhythmia	Cats: cleaning products

Symptoms	Possible Sources
Central nervous system depression/ dysfunction	Birds: cleaning products; lead Cats: cleaning products; lead Dogs: cleaning products; lead
Chomping of jaws	Dogs: lead
Colic	Cats: cleaning products; pesticides and flea repellents Dogs: cleaning products; lead; pesticides and flea repellents
Collapse	Birds: carbon monoxide Cats: carbon monoxide Dogs: carbon monoxide
Coma	Birds: carbon monoxide Cats: carbon monoxide; cleaning products Dogs: carbon monoxide; cleaning products
Confusion	Birds: carbon monoxide Cats: carbon monoxide Dogs: carbon monoxide
Convulsions	Birds: carbon monoxide Cats: carbon monoxide; lead; pesticides and flea repellents; toxic plants Dogs: carbon monoxide; lead; pesticides and flea repellents; toxic plants
Corneal damage	Birds: cleaning products Cats: cleaning products Dogs: cleaning products

Symptoms	Possible Sources
Cough	Birds: building and decorating materials; cleaning products; mold, dust
	Cats: building and decorating materials; cleaning products; mold, dust
	Dogs: building and decorating materials; cleaning products; mold, dust
	(For solutions to mold and dust, see "Healthy Air," Chapter 8.)
Dental fluorosis (staining of the teeth)	Cats: contaminated water
	Dogs: contaminated water
Depression	Birds: building and decorating materials; lack of sunlight
	Cats: building and decorating materials; pesticides and flea repellents; lack of sunlight
	Dogs: building and decorating materials; pesticides and flea repellents; lack of sunlight
	(For a solution to illness-provoking lack of sunlight, see "Indoor Lighting," under "Solutions," Chapter 1.)
Diarrhea	Cats: cleaning products; pesticides and flea repellents
	Dogs: cleaning products; lead; pesticides and flea repellents
Distemper-like behavior	Dogs: contaminated water
Drooping wings	Birds: pesticides
Eczema	Cats: contaminated water
	Dogs: contaminated water

Symptoms	Possible Sources
Erratic flight	Birds: pesticides
Excessive salivation	Cats: cleaning products; toxic plants Dogs: cleaning products; toxic plants
Foaming at the mouth	Cats: cleaning products; pesticides and flea repellents Dogs: cleaning products; pesticides and flea repellents
Gastric upset	Cats: lead; contaminated water Dogs: contaminated water
Gastroenteritis	Cats: pesticides and flea repellents; toxic plants Dogs: pesticides and flea repellents; toxic plants
Hair loss	Cats: cleaning products
Head tremors	Birds: pesticides
Heart action depression	Birds: carbon monoxide Cats: carbon monoxide Dogs: carbon monoxide
Hormonal changes	Birds: building and decorating materials; cleaning products; pesticides; contaminated water Cats: building and decorating materials; cleaning products; pesticides; contaminated water Dogs: building and decorating materials; cleaning products; pesticides; contaminated water

Symptoms	Possible Sources
Hyperactivity	Cats: cleaning products
Hyperthermia	Cats: cleaning products
	Dogs: cleaning products
Hysteria	Cats: lead
Increased respiratory rate	Cats: pesticides and flea repellents
	Dogs: pesticides and flea repellents
Indiscriminate biting	Dogs: lead
Infertility problems	Cats: pesticides and flea repellents
	Dogs: pesticides and flea repellents
Irritability	Birds: building and decorating materials; carbon monoxide
	Cats: building and decorating materials; carbon monoxide; pesticides and flea repellents
	Dogs: building and decorating materials; carbon monoxide; pesticides and flea repellents
Kidney problems	Cats: lead
	Dogs: lead
Listlessness	Birds: pesticides
Mouth and lip irritation	Cats: toxic plants
	Dogs: toxic plants

Symptoms	Possible Sources
Muscle spasms	Birds: lead
Muscle weakness	Cats: cleaning products; pesticides and flea repellents
	Dogs: cleaning products; pesticides and flea repellents
Nausea	Birds: building and decorating materials; carbon monoxide
	Cats: building and decorating materials; carbon monoxide; pesticides and flea repellents; toxic plants; contaminated water
	Dogs: building and decorating materials; carbon monoxide; pesticides and flea repellents; toxic plants; contaminated water
Nervousness	Birds: building and decorating materials
	Cats: building and decorating materials; pesticides and flea repellents
	Dogs: building and decorating materials; pesticides and flea repellents
Neurological disorders	Birds: lead; contaminated water
	Cats: lead; contaminated water
	Dogs: lead; contaminated water
Panting	Cats: cleaning products
Paralysis	Birds: pesticides
Regurgitation	Birds: pesticides

Symptoms	Possible Sources
Reproductive disorders (including infertility and sexual organ deformity)	Birds: lead; pesticides Cats: lead; pesticides and flea repellents Dogs: lead; pesticides and flea repellents
Respiratory stress and possibly failure	Birds: carbon monoxide; cleaning products Cats: carbon monoxide; cleaning products; pesticides Dogs: carbon monoxide; cleaning products; pesticides
Restlessness	Birds: cleaning products; contaminated water Cats: cleaning products; contaminated water Dogs: cleaning products; lead; contaminated water
Ruffled feathers	Birds: pesticides
Seizures	Birds: cleaning products Cats: cleaning products; pesticides and flea repellents Dogs: cleaning products; pesticides and flea repellents
Sexual organ deformity	Cats: pesticides and flea repellents Dogs: pesticides and flea repellents
Shallow breathing	Cats: cleaning products Dogs: cleaning products

Symptoms	Possible Sources
Shock	Cats: cleaning products
Shortness of breath	Birds: carbon monoxide; pesticides Cats: carbon monoxide Dogs: carbon monoxide
Side-to-side head movements	Birds: pesticides
Skin rash (*see also* skin ulcers)	Birds: building and decorating materials Cats: building and decorating materials; contaminated water Dogs: building and decorating materials; contaminated water
Skin ulcers	Cats: cleaning products Dogs: cleaning products
Slow respiration	Cats: cleaning products Dogs: cleaning products
Stiffness	Cats: pesticides Dogs: pesticides
Swallowing difficulty	Cats: toxic plants Dogs: toxic plants
Vomiting (*see also* regurgitation)	Birds: carbon monoxide; pesticides; contaminated water Cats: carbon monoxide; cleaning products; pesticides and flea repellents; toxic plants; contaminated water

Symptoms	Possible Sources
	Dogs: carbon monoxide; cleaning products; lead; pesticides and flea repellents; toxic plants; contaminated water
Watery eyes and nose	Cats: toxic plants Dogs: toxic plants
Weakness	Cats: pesticides and flea repellents Dogs: pesticides and flea repellents
Whining/ growling	Dogs: lead

1.
Building and Decorating Dangers

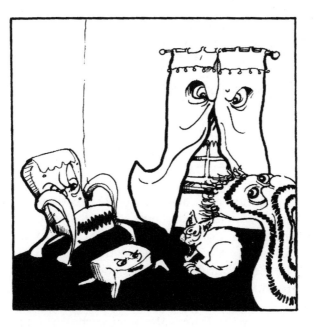

G randma used to say, "Everything is safe in moderation." Unfortunately, we do not breathe indoor air in moderation, and far too much of it is toxic for both pets and humans. Even moderate amounts of chemical inhalation can cause a lifetime of sickness. Ironically, the places where we feel safest—our homes—often contain building and decorating materials that pollute our air and put our health at great risk. And since most pets spend much of their time inside the house, they are closer to toxic sources for longer periods of time than we are. Furthermore, they inhale higher concentrations of poisonous chemicals for their given body weights. Therefore, many symptoms attributed to poisonous fumes can appear in our animals before they appear in us.

The Problem

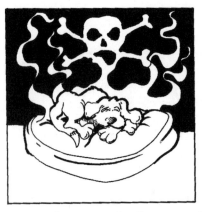

It is only in recent years that indoor building and decorating materials have been considered hazardous. Many of these products contain a variety of harmful adhesives, plastics, fire-retardant sprays, and/or paints containing volatile organic compounds (VOCs). Such substances release—or *outgas*—dangerous fumes that accumulate inside houses that lack good ventilation. Modern insulation methods contribute greatly to this lack of air exchange; function has been so perfected that air does not leak into or out of the structure. Captured within these "tight houses" are also mold spores that lurk in damp areas, heating systems, humidifiers, carpets, and dust. And such homes are more likely to contain lethal amounts of carbon monoxide—a noxious gas that escapes from faulty heating systems. (For more information on carbon monoxide, see Chapter 2.)

This chapter discusses the harmful results of extensive exposure to the following: formaldehyde; indoor lighting; plastics; synthetic carpet toxins; and volatile organic compounds (VOCs) found in paint and other household materials. It then offers several suggestions on how to reduce and/or remove these building and decorating hazards.

Symptoms Resulting from Hazardous Building and Decorating Materials

As is the case with most environmental pollutants, the symptoms produced by harmful building and decorating materials will vary, depending on the type of substance that is causing the problem. However, there are several general indications for which to watch. The following apply to birds, cats, and dogs:

- Anxiety
- Breathing problems
- Cancer
- Cough
- Depression
- Hormonal changes
- Irritability
- Nausea
- Nervousness
- Skin rash

Formaldehyde

Formaldehyde is found in many products, including glue, adhesives, paint preservatives, pressed-wood products, fabric finishes, paneling, and ventless fuel-burning appliances. Your pet can be poisoned by formaldehyde fumes if you keep him or her in a tightly closed house that lacks proper air circulation and ventilation. In addition to the above-mentioned sources, many sofas, draperies, and bedding materials have formaldehyde-based finishes, such as permanent press and stain-resistant coatings. Any pet that sleeps on these surfaces can be affected. Remember that cats and dogs sleep longer and more often than people do. If their beds or sleeping places have chemicals in the fabric, they will experience heavy exposure to toxins.

People who have been harmed by formaldehyde fumes often exhibit the following symptoms: watery eyes; sore throat; nausea; skin rash; cough; fatigue; excessive thirst; nosebleeds; and difficulty breathing. Pets react similarly. In addition, formaldehyde has been proven to cause cancer in animals. If you recently have redecorated and your pet exhibits any of the symptoms listed on page 15, consider that formaldehyde poisoning may be the culprit. Keep in mind that outgassing fumes are at their strongest when building or decorating materials are new. In addition, high indoor temperatures and humidity levels cause the release of these gases to increase.

Indoor Lighting

You may not think of light as a pollutant but, in some ways, it is. While exposure to artificial lighting does not cause physical sickness, a lack of full-spectrum light can trigger extreme mood swings and depression, causing an illness known as *seasonal affective disorder* (SAD). Both humans and pets suffer from this illness.

During the winter months, your animal may become lethargic, have a greater appetite, and put on weight. This could be due to a lack of natural light. Sunlight emits a complete spectrum, whereas conventional indoor illumination emits an overabundance of yellow light. The absence of a balanced spectrum promotes anxiety, depression, fatigue, and irritability. If your pet is outside for a good portion of the day, he or she probably will not experience this disorder. However, pets who are generally confined to indoor lighting environments are susceptible to SAD. An animal's body needs sunlight to stimulate essential biological functions. Furthermore, artificial lighting affects menstrual regularity and fertility in animals, as its unchanging brightness causes the irregular release of the hormone *melatonin*.

Plastics

The plastics industry continues to thrive, despite a growing awareness of the toxins that plastics produce. The harm comes from the outgassing of minute quantities of toxic vapors. These fumes can have a cumulative effect on the body, causing disease when concentrations rise to high levels. The following materials are some of the substances from which noxious vapors are released: polyvinyl chloride (PVC), found in pipes; polyurethane resin, contained in glues and in pillow foams; urea-formaldehyde resin, commonly used in insulation and foam cushions; plasticizers—substances that are added to plastics and other materials to maintain pliability; and synthetic rubbers.

Synthetic Carpet Toxins

The number of cases concerning the harmful effects of new synthetic carpets is rising. Even the Environmental Protection Agency experienced a problem with toxic carpeting. In 1987, the agency installed 27,000 yards of carpet in one of their office complexes. Eighteen months later, after scores of complaints and reported illnesses from the workers, the carpet was removed. Although the EPA maintained that no scientific evidence linked the carpeting to the workers' health problems, the action to remove the carpet spoke for itself.

In the past, most manufacturers of synthetic carpets used a glue called *4-PC* to affix the carpet backing. This glue has been proven to be highly toxic. Fortunately, many companies are eliminating the use of 4-PC, but you should read the label on the carpet to be sure this adhesive has not been applied. Some of the many other dangerous chemicals found in synthetic carpets include formaldehyde, toluene, xylene, tetrachloroethylene, styrene, ethylbenzene, and phthalic esters. All of these substances can make your pet sick. Animals who spend most of their time on the floor, at the source of the poisonous chemicals, are much more susceptible to these toxins than we are.

Synthetic carpet fumes produce numerous symptoms in humans, including burning eyes, chills, sore throat, cough, nausea, dizziness, nervousness, and depression. If your pet could talk, he or she might complain of the same symptoms. Since it is difficult to determine if your animal companion has burning eyes or a sore throat, you should carefully watch his or her behavior, especially if you recently installed a new synthetic carpet.

Volatile Organic Compounds (VOCs)

No one considered paint a harmful substance until it was discovered that lead, one of its long-time ingredients, causes illness, especially in children. (For more information on lead poisoning, see Chapter 4.) Lead paint was outlawed in 1978, and we thought we were safe until more research found another culprit: volatile organic compounds (VOCs)—chemically unstable organic compounds that exist in liquid or solid form and, if combined with other chemicals, may cause dangerous reactions when inhaled or absorbed through the skin. These toxins, some of which are benzene, methylene chloride, and perchloroethylene, contribute to smog and ozone pollution. They also pollute our indoor environments, putting pets and owners at risk.

VOCs are common ingredients in paints, varnishes, solvents, stains, strippers, all-purpose cleaners, de-greasing and hobby products, moth repellents, and air fresheners. Some of the many common household VOC vapors are: acetone, in nail polish, tobacco smoke, and paint thinner; benzene, in adhesives, spot cleaners, and particle board; chlorobenzene, in DDT and paint thinner; ethylbenzene, in floor and wall coverings; styrene, in uretheyne foam insulation; toluene, in adhesives, paint, washable wallpaper, and plastic flooring; tri-chloroethylene, in paint thinner; and xylene, in adhesives, flooring, and wallpaper.

Side effects that result from exposure to these fumes include respiratory irritation, kidney problems, asthma, wheezing, and croup (a laryngeal condition, especially affecting the young, that involves respiratory ailments and a severe cough). Animals suffer from additional symptoms that are more difficult to diagnose, such as visual disorders, depression, and memory impairment. Furthermore, VOCs have been proven to cause cancer in animals. And in "A Guide to Indoor Air Quality," published in 1988 by the U.S. Consumer Product Safety Commission, the Environmental Protection Agency reports that many of these organic pollutants are five times more concentrated inside our buildings, as compared with outside.

VOCs can also be found in water. Landfill and industrial waste pollution seeps into our ground water. The compounds rapidly evaporate into the air during normal household activities such as washing dishes, doing the laundry, flushing the toilet, and taking a shower.

The Solution

The most obvious solution to chemical pollution is to go back to nature and live without toxic materials. Unfortunately, this is neither practical nor possible. Steps are being taken, however, to encourage less hazardous living environments. Manufacturers are beginning to create safer building and decorating materials, either because they recognize the dangers of their product ingredients or because they are required to comply with new laws. Still, it is close to impossible to find current building products that are chemical-free. So we must find solutions that work from within the home.

Air circulation is fundamental to reducing the poisonous threat of every toxin discussed in this chapter. Today, heating costs are so high that most people don't want to open windows and let the heat escape. As a result, homes become toxic gas chambers. If you are adamant about keeping your house tightly shut, consider installing a heat-recovery ventilation system or an air-circulation fan system, both of which exchange the air many times within each hour. Clean air is essential to your pet's health, as well as to your own. If your pet develops an illness because of "sick building" syndrome, the rest of your family will surely follow.

Formaldehyde

There are home-test kits available to determine the level of formaldehyde in your house, but the methods used in home-test canisters often do not provide accurate measurements. If you suspect a problem, have a professional lab perform the evaluation.

Types of Air Treatment Units

Many air treatment units are effective at removing poisonous gasses, zapping pollutants out of the air, and keeping mold at bay. One type of device uses natural ozone combined with a negative ionizer. The ozone attaches to airborne particles and converts them to harmless compounds that fall to the floor or dissipate. The negative ions promote a sense of well-being in animals (including us). Birds stop picking their feathers and dogs stop scratching because the purification device reduces the amount of allergic contamination in the air. This type of unit is highly effective for reducing allergies in kennels and aviaries, and for improving your pet's state of mind.

Electrostatic units use both negative and positive ions to attract contaminants to the air-cleaner unit, where they are caught in a removable filter. Other air treatment systems use sophisticated HEPA (high-efficiency particulate arrestor) and carbon filters to clean gas and particulate from the air. Information on specific brands of air treatment devices is given in the Product Directory (page 117). You should analyze your specific needs and choose a unit that is specific to that application.

Alternatives to formaldehyde-based products are available: solid wood furniture; natural cotton bedding and fabric coverings; natural carpets made of nontoxic wool, jute, or sisal; and hardwood flooring. For a simple and immediate solution, you can purchase an air treatment device to purify poisonous fumes. (See "Types of Air Treatment Units," above.)

Indoor Lighting

A simple solution to your pet's extended exposure to artificial lighting is the installation of full-spectrum light bulbs, commonly known as *plant lights*. These bulbs mimic daylight and should raise your pet's spirits. Zoos have reported that birds, fish, and other animals show improvements in their health when simu-

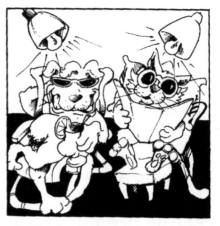

lated sunlight is introduced. Chicken farmers discovered that when they installed full-spectrum lights, the birds acted less aggressively, the cholesterol content of their eggs was reduced, and their productive life was lengthened. Full-spectrum lights are listed in the Product Directory.

Plastics

To avoid outgassing fumes from plastic-based furniture, flooring, storage containers, and so on, investigate more natural alternatives and be sure to read labels. Purchase wood or metal items that are finished with nontoxic paint. Install hardwood instead of particle board flooring; ceramic tile instead of formica; and, for insulation, expanded polystyrene only. When applying glues, do so in a well-ventilated area that is not located near your living space, and let the materials outgas for several months before bringing them into the house. Do not store plastic outdoor furniture, glues, or resins inside or near your dwelling, as fumes from these items will be poisonous to your pets, your family, and you.

Synthetic Carpet Toxins

Synthetic carpet manufacturers comply with a limit for toxic emissions and may indicate safer carpets on the labels. However, the safest alternative is to purchase nontoxic wool, jute, or sisal carpets. Natural-fiber carpets have always been available, but it has been only in the last few years that they have become competitive in price. Hardwood floors are also an option.

If your carpet contains toxins but you cannot remove it, consider purchasing an air treatment device that can effectively eliminate the fumes. You can also apply nontoxic sprays that lock in the toxins and reduce their emissions.

Volatile Organic Compounds (VOCs)

The obvious way to protect your pet and yourself from inadvertent VOC-poisoning is to reduce (as much as possible) your use of products that contain volatile organic compounds. Low-VOC paint has appeared on the commercial market, in addition to already established "natural" paints. Nontoxic paints, strippers, and solvents are widely available from catalogs, eco-stores, and some retail paint outlets. Please be aware that while low-VOC paints are less toxic than regular paints when inhaled, they are lethal if your pet drinks them. It is important to keep *all* decorating and cleaning products away from your pet.

Other ways to reduce or eliminate VOCs include using cedar shavings instead of mothballs; replacing chemical all-purpose cleaning products with baking soda or with vinegar and salt; and purchasing natural (non-chemical) air fresheners found in health food stores. Air purification devices also aid in the reduction of VOCs.

As discussed earlier, VOCs contaminate the water supply as well. Toxins generally accumulate on the surface of the liquid—a process called *adsorption*. Point-of-use carbon filters, which are easily installed, effectively remove these toxins from the water. Be sure to properly maintain and frequently change the filter.

While you are considering the dangerous impact of building and decorating materials that are used in construction and home maintenance, also keep in mind the toxic properties of the common office and art supplies that are often left on top of desks and on open shelves: glues, correction fluid, toner, pens, paints, solvents, crayons, clay, and other craft materials. These substances will cause illness if eaten or licked by your pet. Children are often taught not to put anything other than food in their mouths. Unfortunately, animals rarely learn this lesson and can become very sick from household items. These materials must be kept out of your pet's reach.

There is light at the end of the tunnel, and it starts with education. Remember, you unknowingly may be creating a toxic chamber for your animal. An indoor pet spends a much greater amount of time in the domicile than you do, and will feel the effects of chemical air pollution far more quickly. Therefore, it is important to be aware of symptoms and causes. With this information, you can evaluate your pet's environment and make your home a safer, healthier place.

2.
Carbon Monoxide–
A Noxious Gas

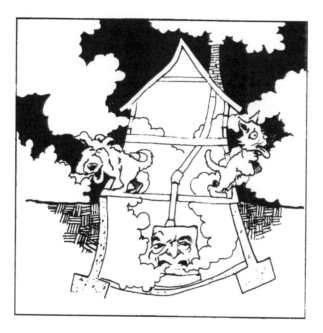

I
t is a pet owner's nightmare to come home to a dead dog, cat, or bird, especially when the animal wasn't sick. Carbon monoxide (CO) can permanently put your pet to sleep without any warning signs. This colorless and odorless gas interferes with the delivery of oxygen to cells in the body. It should not be confused with carbon dioxide, a relatively harmless gas that can be found, for example, in the

bubbles in soft drinks. Carbon monoxide kills people as well as animals, so if your pet has died in the house unexpectedly, you should investigate carbon monoxide poisoning for your own safety. Better yet, read this chapter carefully and seek prevention before *any* harm is done.

The Problem

When carbon monoxide enters the bloodstream, it replaces normal oxygen-carrying hemoglobin with carboxyhemoglobin (COHb)—a compound that prevents life-supporting oxygen from reaching the heart, brain, and other body organs. Carbon monoxide may cause permanent brain damage, resulting in personality changes and loss of memory in humans. It can also be deadly. Fatal CO levels depend on an animal's size and the length of exposure time. Birds can die from very low levels of carbon monoxide if their cages are kept close to faulty gas stoves or heaters.

Carbon monoxide poisoning is a growing problem. Many of our modern combustion appliances, such as furnaces, gas stoves, and space heaters, can emit carbon monoxide if they are not functioning properly. Because today's homes are built to be airtight, gasses are unable to escape and toxins build to dangerous concentrations. As mentioned previously, carbon monoxide does not have an odor or a color. Without a special carbon monoxide detector, it is impossible to gauge this hazard until inhabitants actually get sick. Even then, carbon monoxide poisoning is often mistaken for the flu. If the CO source is not identified and fixed, the gas will accumulate to potentially lethal levels.

"Combustion Appliances and Indoor Air Pollution," published in 1991 by the US Consumer Product Safety Commission, reports statistics showing that nearly 300 human deaths per year are caused by carbon monoxide released from fuel-burning appliances (not fires). One can only guess how many pets lose their lives for the same reason. The winter months are especially dangerous, since closed windows trap lethal amounts of carbon monoxide inside the

Symptoms of Carbon Monoxide Poisoning

Birds, cats, and dogs suffer the same symptoms of carbon monoxide poisoning. These include:

- Collapse
- Coma
- Confusion
- Convulsion
- Heart action depression
- Irritability
- Nausea
- Respiratory stress and possible failure
- Shortness of breath
- Vomiting

Carbon monoxide is a deadly gas. If exposure continues, the next occurrence is death. For information on the progression of symptoms according to the level of carboxyhemoglobin in the blood, see "Dangerous Accumulations" (page 28).

house. Unfortunately, this dangerous gas usually claims victims while they sleep.

In humans, carbon monoxide poisoning can cause flu-like symptoms, shortness of breath, hyper-irritability, dizziness, headaches, nausea, confusion, disorientation, and fatigue. Exposure to high concentrations of carbon monoxide for as little as two hours can result in unconsciousness and death. See "Are You Poisoning Yourself?" (page 29) for more information on the warning signs of carbon monoxide poisoning in the human body. If you notice any of these symptoms, check your carbon monoxide detector, call a professional service person, and remove yourself and your pet from the house until the problem is fixed.

Sources of Carbon Monoxide

Carbon monoxide can accumulate in any place where combustion appliances are used. The most common area of risk

Dangerous Accumulations

The following table shows the effects that different blood levels of carbon monoxide have on animals. The percentage of carboxyhemoglobin (COHb) indicates the amount of carbon monoxide in the blood.

% Carboxyhemoglobin (COHb) in the Blood	Symptoms
10% COHb	No signs
10%–20% COHb	Shortness of breath during moderate exercise
30% COHb	Hyper-irritability, nausea, vomiting
40% COHb	Confusion, collapse, coma
50%–60% COHb	Respiratory failure, coma, convulsions
60%–70% COHb	Coma, convulsions, depressed heart action, death
70%–80% COHb	Death within hours
80%–90% COHb	Death in less than an hour
90%+ COHb	Death in minutes

in the home is a closed garage in which automobiles are left running. The resulting build-up of gas becomes deadly within a relatively short amount of time. Other sources include gas and oil furnaces, fireplaces and wood-burning stoves, gas appliances such as stoves and dryers, gas or kerosene space heaters, and indoor charcoal grills.

Are You Poisoning Yourself?

If you think carbon monoxide is affecting your pet, it also may be affecting you. Ask yourself the following questions:

☐ Do you feel unusually sleepy?

☐ Do you have headaches, dizziness, or nausea?

☐ Do you have watery eyes and feel nose or throat irritation without having a cold or other known illness?

☐ Do the symptoms occur only in your house or office?

☐ Do the symptoms disappear after you have left the house or office for a while?

☐ Does anyone else in the house or office have these symptoms?

☐ Have you recently had more cases of the flu than usual?

☐ Are your symptoms getting worse?

If your answer to any of these questions is "yes," you might have carbon monoxide poisoning, and so might your pet.

Unlike many pets, people have the opportunity to leave the house during the day, so unless the carbon monoxide is at high concentrations, you are not likely to be affected. However, some symptoms could still appear, such as sniffles, fatigue, and difficulty concentrating while in the house. If these symptoms disappear when you leave your home, suspect carbon monoxide and remove your pet from the house until you have absolutely determined that carbon monoxide levels are not dangerous.

Houses that have been built in compliance with the new insulation standards have few air leaks. As a result of poor ventilation, the furnace does not get the air it needs to operate properly. It creates negative pressure, sucking carbon monoxide fumes into the home from the furnace exhaust pipe, which is located in or near the fireplace or chimney. A pet who is left indoors could die from the accumulation of this noxious gas.

If your home is heated by a forced hot air furnace, be wary of leaks in the piping. These leaks may cause gas to spread more quickly into the house through the hot air ducts. Electric heating systems are much less risky; if your water heater and appliances are electric, you most likely do not have to worry about carbon monoxide seeping from these sources. Do not use gas or kerosene space heaters to augment electric heat unless they are working properly and are placed in well-ventilated areas.

Fireplaces and wood-burning stoves can emit carbon monoxide if the wood is not burning completely and if the flues are clogged or improperly installed. It is advisable for homes that use fireplaces or wood stoves to have a carbon monoxide detector on hand. Also, using a charcoal grill indoors is extremely dangerous, as this type of appliance is a hazardous CO source. Finally, common household chemicals can be responsible for carbon monoxide poisoning. Some paint removers and solvents, for example, contain methylene chloride, which releases fumes that change to carbon monoxide.

The Solution

If you suspect your pet's symptoms are caused by carbon monoxide, immediately open windows and doors, shut off appliances, and take your pet outdoors. Contact a veterinarian right away and tell him or her why you suspect carbon monoxide poisoning. (Examine yourself for symptoms, as well.) A veterinarian can diagnose carbon monoxide poisoning by means of a blood test that measures the blood level of CO combined with hemoglobin. Because CO leaves the blood slowly, this test can identify the problem even if the blood specimen is taken one or two hours after you have left the suspected environment. If test results indicate the presence of carbon monoxide in your pet's body, you immediately should locate the source in your home, rectify the problem, and prevent CO from further poisoning your family.

Detecting Carbon Monoxide in Your Home

Carbon monoxide detector kits are inexpensive and easy to use. Each kit provides a colormetric disk that affixes to any area in your home. The disk changes color if carbon monoxide is present, and the time it takes to turn color indicates the severity of the CO level. For example, it took fifteen to forty-five minutes for 100 parts per million (ppm) of carbon monoxide to register on the disks of the test-kits that we tried. When we increased the CO level to 600 ppm, the disks indicated the presence of carbon monoxide within one to two minutes. Damp weather may increase the test-kits' reaction times, while dry weather may slow the process down. *Any* indication of carbon monoxide should be taken seriously.

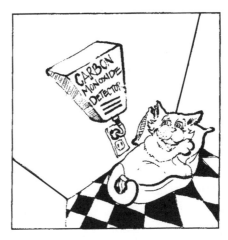

It is best to install the colormetric detectors in several rooms. Check them several times a day to see if any changes have taken place. Often, people install the detector, determine that their home is safe on one day, and don't check again. However, appliances can have faulty systems that suddenly break down, so daily and repeated monitoring is best.

A more reliable alternative to the colormetric disk test is an electrically operated carbon monoxide detector that sounds an alarm if the gas is present. This device, similar to an automatic smoke alarm, does not require daily checking. You should install one of these units on each floor of your house. Many states are considering legislation that would make these detectors mandatory in certain types of housing. In fact, the city of Chicago has already implemented requirements for carbon monoxide detectors.

Preventing Carbon Monoxide Poisoning

Proper ventilation is essential for the reduction of any fire- or fuel-burning appliance hazard. Opening a window and running exhaust fans can help, but this will raise your heating bills. Heat recovery ventilators—machines that bring fresh air into and draw stale air out of the home—can do the job with minimal heat loss, but installation is difficult unless you are building a new structure or have an existing forced hot air system. The most practical solution is to keep existing vents and ducts clear, to service your appliances regularly, and to purchase a CO detection device.

The most important part of preparing for the winter season is to have a professional service person clean your furnace and secure that the flame is adjusted to maintain a clean burn. Have the heat box checked for cracks and make repairs, if necessary. Confirm that there is an adequate air supply to and around the furnace, preferably ducting air from the outdoors. Prior to turning on the heat, hire a service to clean any forced hot air ducts that you may have. You can clean the flue yourself, if maintenance personnel are not available. Also, be sure to change the furnace filter often.

While the furnace is on, frequently check the flame to insure a complete burn. The flame should be blue. A yellow flame indicates that the burner must be adjusted; the yellow color is due to the presence of carbon, which produces carbon monoxide. If you smell fuel, suspect a problem and call a maintenance person. Finally, make sure that all panels and grills are in place, and that the fan door is closed when the furnace is operating.

Furnaces made after 1982 are required to have a pilot light safety system called an *oxygen depletion sensor* (ODS). This feature shuts off the heater when there is not enough fresh air to have an effective burn. Another type of safety measure is available in gas appliances that are installed with electronic ignitions, as these avoid the problem of continuous low-level pollutants being released from pilot lights. No furnace is guaranteed to prevent carbon monoxide from entering the house, but with proper maintenance, your furnace should work as designed and not pose a hazard.

As previously discussed, your fireplace is another area of possible danger. Clean the flue and chimney each autumn. Whenever a wood-burning stove or fireplace is in operation, maintain good ventilation by leaving the flue open. As fire prevention requires, be sure the fire is out before you go to sleep.

If you use a space heater that is fueled by a combustible material such as kerosene, adequate ventilation is absolutely necessary. This not only keeps the unit burning efficiently, therefore emitting less carbon monoxide, but also protects you from any harmful concentrations of gas build-up. When using these supplemental heaters, you should always have a carbon monoxide detector in the house.

Finally, we have a few more pointers. Never run your car in a closed garage that is attached to the house. Fumes from the exhaust can be drawn into the home and can remain there for a period of time, especially if the house is well-insulated. Never use outdoor barbecue grills in a closed room, unless the grill is vented to the outside. Many people and pets have been fatally poisoned by carbon monoxide released during the indoor use of a charcoal grill. Concerning chemical CO sources, always ensure proper air ventilation when chemical substances are being applied, and use nontoxic, natural products, where possible.

Considering the various devices and services available today, there is no reason why anyone, pets included, should be harmed by carbon monoxide. Install carbon monoxide detectors or alarms, frequently check the condition of your combustion appliances, and watch for any symptoms—in your pet and in yourself—that may arise. Know the signs of CO poisoning before levels rise to a lethal dose. Lastly, since animals who are home alone can't save themselves when an alarm sounds, be extremely prudent; avoid risky appliances. You and your pet are safest when you take the necessary measures to *prevent* CO poisoning.

3.
Cleaners That Kill

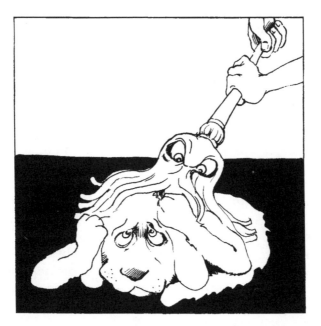

M ost of us are highly concerned with keeping our living spaces clean. Household cupboards are filled with floor cleaners, carpet cleaners and deodorizers, tile cleaners, drain cleaners, air fresheners, stain-resistant sprays, spot removers, waxes, abrasives, bleaches, and soaps. The manufacturers of these products warn us not to ingest the substances and not to allow them to come into contact with our eyes. Labels include instructions to use the substances only in well-ventilated places. We know that these products are toxic, but may not be able to determine *how* toxic because the ingredients are either not listed or incomprehensible. Thus, it is easy to clean, polish, and leave the house, never realizing that indoor pets are left behind in a poisonous environment.

The Problem

Pets are more susceptible to hazardous cleaning products than humans because they spend most of their time on the floor, where fumes are strongest. Animals may walk over freshly washed or waxed floors and then lick the cleaner off their paws. Toxins from flea repellents, carpet fresheners, and spot cleaners pervade carpeting and can attach to pets' fur. Aerosol sprays are also a hazard to an animal's health, especially if the pet already has respiratory problems. And those pleasantly scented air fresheners, which are fatal if eaten, are laden with chemicals that permeate the indoor environment. Fumes left over from these and other cleaning products can linger in the home for long periods of time, particularly when the windows are closed during the heating and air conditioning seasons.

Concerns about cleaning product poisoning constituted 4 percent of all calls to the Illinois Animal Poison Information Center in 1987. Distressed pet owners asked questions about general cleaners, bath and tile cleaners, floor and wall cleaners, industrial cleaners, dishwashing detergents, bleaches, corrosives, disinfectants, carpet products, and laundry products. Approximately 85 percent of these calls involved accidental exposure in the home, mostly concerning oral ingestion. Dogs are more likely to ingest toxic substances than cats, because dogs will put just about anything in their mouths.

The chemicals in many household cleaners can cause genetic damage to pets. Most of the applicable animal studies have determined that the ingestion of toxic levels of chemicals can cause cancer, but only recently have scientists begun to study the effects of these contaminants on reproduction. Hormonal pollutants, which are breakdown products of common detergents, have been found to cause increased levels of estrogen—a female hormone—in male animals. This can have widespread consequences, for although you may not notice the effect in your spayed or neutered pet, such a process could result in the demise of many species of wildlife. Modern lifestyles have far-reaching ramifications, and what is washed down the sinks and released into the air could poison countless families and pets, as well as the natural environment. Please be responsible and consider all of the implications of your actions when you go shopping for household products.

Detergents and Disinfectants

Pets are exposed to soap, laundry, and deodorizer product toxins in a variety of ways, some of which are: ingesting soap bars; rooting around the laundry room soap boxes; walking on recently washed or waxed floors; and inhaling deodorizer sprays. Commercial bar soaps are the most com-

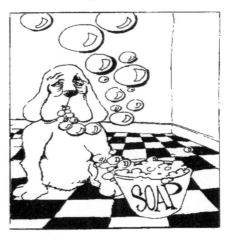

mon source of toxicity in animals, but, luckily, they induce reactions that are usually not fatal. The ingestion of soap can cause vomiting and diarrhea, possibly due to the essential oils and chemical fragrances. These symptoms disrupt the animal's electrolyte balance, which is essential to maintaining the body's healthy life-force.

According to "Laundry Detergents," an article in the Washington Toxic Coalition's *Alternative Fact Sheet* (October, 1992), most detergents can be categorized as nonionic or

Symptoms of Cleaning Product Poisoning

While the actual symptoms of cleaning product poisoning that an animal exhibits depend on the type of substance to which he or she was exposed, there are some general symptoms of which you should be aware. For dogs and cats, these include:

- Anxiety
- Burns on the mouth and esophagus
- Central nervous system depression
- Colic
- Coma
- Corneal damage
- Cough
- Diarrhea
- Excessive salivation
- Foaming at the mouth
- Hormonal changes
- Hyperthermia
- Muscle weakness
- Restlessness
- Seizures
- Shallow breathing
- Skin ulcers
- Slow respiration
- Vomiting

In addition to the above-listed symptoms, cats, who can have fatal reactions to cleaning products, also experience the following:

- Cardiac arrhythmia
- Hair loss
- Hyperactivity
- Panting
- Shock

Birds who have been poisoned by cleaning products suffer from:

- Anxiety
- Breathing problems
- Corneal damage
- Cough
- Hormonal changes
- Seizures

anionic, and both types are toxic. Nonionic (neutrally charged) synthetic detergents found in dishwashing liquids and shampoos include alkyl ethoxylate, alkyl phenoxy poly-ethoxy ethanol, and polyethylene glycol stearate. Anionic (negatively charged) detergents commonly found in laundry products contain alkyl sodium sulfates, alkyl sodium sulfonates, dioctyl sodium sulfosuccinate, sodium lauryl sulfates, tetrapropylene benzene sulfonates, and linear alkyl benzene sulfonates. Animals exposed to these above-named ingredients will suffer from vomiting and diarrhea. It is important to store laundry detergents in a place that is inaccessible to your pet.

Unless it is broken, your pet's skin will provide a good external barrier and protect the animal from the toxic effects of most detergents. If the detergent comes into contact with your pet's eyes, however, corneal damage is a strong possibility. It is very important to call a poison control center immediately. Every household should have the telephone number of a poison control center posted on or next to the telephone because, in an emergency, every moment counts. Please see the Information Resources list, page 115, for the phone number of the National Animal Poison Control Center.

If a detergent is ingested, it is likely to be metabolized by the liver and excreted in the urine, but there have been cases of permanently impaired liver function due to certain concentrations of detergent in the blood. Even if the toxins are excreted through the urine, your pet may still experience diarrhea and vomiting. Therefore, it is best to use biodegradable soaps that contain the least amount of toxic products as possible. Though it requires some research and self-education, reading labels and comparing ingredients is important. And after all, your pet's health is worth it.

Fabric softeners, germicides, and sanitizers are capable of burning your animal's mouth and esophagus, as well as damaging mucous membranes. These products can also cause excessive salivation; corneal damage; vomiting; muscle weakness; central nervous system depression; skin ulcers; seizures; coma; and death. Hair loss is another common symptom for cats who have been poisoned by these products.

Disinfectant cleaners usually contain more than one of the following chemicals: creosol; phenol; formaldehyde; ammonia; chlorine; and ethanol. Because of the reactions that occur between these chemicals, toxic effects worsen. Cats are especially susceptible to products containing phenols, which, if ingested, can result in burns of the mouth and esophagus, vomiting, excessive salivation, apprehension, hyperactivity, and panting. This toxicity can progress to include shock, cardiac arrhythmia (a change in heart rhythm), and coma. Pine oil affects cats in a similar manner. If a cat has lapped up this substance, he or she will develop a pine-smelling breath, which will alert you of the situation. In such a case, seek immediate treatment; cats can die within twelve hours if enough pine oil is ingested.

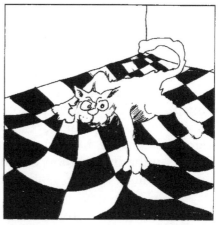

Bleaches cause symptoms similar to those inflicted by phenols and pine oil, although they may not cause illness as rapidly as pine oil. The smell of chlorine-based bleach is usually noticeable on the animal's breath. If your pet inhales fumes from bleach powders, he or she may react by coughing or retching. When chlorine bleach is mixed with ammonia or vinegar, the combination can produce very toxic chloramine fumes. Non-chlorine bleaches such as hydrogen peroxide bleaches, which are generally low in toxicity, are available. These products have been proven to be much safer than chlorine bleaches, but are not harmless; gastritis, or inflammation of the stomach, is associated with the ingestion of non-chlorine bleach. This type of substance, too, should be detectable on your pet's breath. Ultimately, all disinfectants should be kept away from animals. Be aware that dogs tend to chew containers, and that pets, in general, lap up liquids and lick substances off their fur.

Our cleaning culture is fond of using canned sprays that are often aerosols. These are harmful substances known to trigger respiratory stress and asthma in humans. Aerosols affect pets in the same way. They are dangerous products that should be avoided.

Garage and Basement Substances

Almost any product used for heavy cleaning, painting, or servicing of cars is toxic to animals. The most common garage poison is antifreeze, which contains ethylene glycol. This dangerous substance can leak from car radiators or spill when you are refilling the canister in your automobile. Other chemicals found in antifreeze are gasoline, copper, zinc, and lead, all of which are harmful to animals if ingested. Never pour antifreeze on the ground or into a stream, as it is a sweet-tasting liquid and very attractive to animals. This product commonly causes cardiac failure and brain damage in household pets who drink it. Within half an hour to an hour following the ingestion of a toxic dose, dogs show signs of anxiety, nausea, and depression. These symptoms progress to coma and death in six to eighteen hours. If smaller amounts are consumed, the animal may vomit and reduce the concentration of the chemical in its system, but death resulting from this incident could still occur within two weeks.

There is a line of "safe" antifreeze on the market. It contains propylene glycol as its active ingredient. If ingested, this substance does not cause the fatal kidney damage that the more toxic antifreezes do, but it does trigger nervous system dysfunction that leads to coordination problems and possibly seizures. Therefore, treat this new antifreeze as you would any other toxin and keep it away from your pet. Also be aware that propylene glycol is added to some food and skin care products for humans. Take precaution and store such items where your animal cannot reach them or, better yet, avoid them completely.

Both kerosene and fuel oil are highly toxic, producing gastroenteritis, circulatory collapse, depression, convulsions, and coma. And turpentine, another product commonly found in garages and basements, is not only poisonous when swallowed, but also can be absorbed through your pet's skin. Turpentine causes nausea, colic, restlessness, coma, and death due to respiratory failure.

The garage area holds many other poisons, including: creosol; naphthalene (mothballs); paraffin; phenol; toluene and xylene (found in paint and thinners); hexachlorophene (germicidal soap); and pine tar. Ingestion of these substances can lead to excessive salivation, weakness, convulsions, hypothermia, paralysis, and death. All of them are known carcinogens in humans, and may be linked to the increasing number of cancer cases in pets. There is little chance that the fumes from stored toxins will affect your pet, since family animals usually don't spend much time in closed garages. Poisoning more often occurs when animals lick up spills and drips.

The Solution

One way to keep your pet safe from cleaning product poisoning is to use natural-based products. It is important for consumers to realize that, although these safer substances are considerably less toxic, they can still have an adverse effect on pets. All cleaning products should be handled with care and stored properly. When you clean surfaces in your house, allow the substance to dry completely and the fumes to dissipate before your pet comes into contact with the area. It is necessary to keep all cleaning products out of your pet's reach and to dispose of the containers carefully.

Detergents and Disinfectants

As mentioned above, it is best to purchase natural cleaning products. We recommend *Citrasolve, ECOVER,* and *Seventh Generation* brands, which are available in many supermarkets and health food/natural product stores. For more suggestions, see the Product Directory, page 117. Natural cleaning substances usually consist of various combinations of the following: borax; lemon juice; dried kelp; coconut-oil derivatives; baking soda; and salt. You can safely make your own solutions, as well. Borax, baking soda, white vinegar, and lemon juice are effective spot removers. Vinegar works well as a de-greaser and window cleaner, instead of ammonia, and also as a fabric softener. A combination of white vinegar, lemon juice, and olive oil provides a good furniture polish. And mixing salt water and baking soda in an aluminum pot yields an all-natural silver polish.

Baking soda and cornstarch are both great carpet fresheners. Lemon grass or cinnamon sticks can be used as natural air fresheners, and citrus/vegetable extract evaporators are also available. Zeolites—crushed porous rocks—are safe deodorizers for litter boxes, pet houses, and runs. They also eliminate urine odor from carpets and can be used in place of tomato juice for removing skunk scent from your dog. Alternatives to mothballs include cedar shavings, lemon grass, lavender, and rosemary. Putting clothes in the dryer or freezer is another way to eliminate moth larvae.

Many nontoxic cleaners contain citrus oils and are far safer than chemical detergents. Pet shampoos and skin products are usually not risky because they contain well-diluted forms of citrus oils. However, *undiluted* citrus oils, which contain D-limonene and linalool, can be dangerous. They are often found in food additives and flea sprays. Crude citrus oil extract is particularly toxic to cats, who can react with excessive salivation and, depending on the level of exposure, can develop muscle tremors, shivering, and hypothermia (a decrease in body temperature). Most cats recover, but death can occur if the animal becomes totally immersed in the liquid. Yet some flea dip containers actually instruct the user to fully soak the animal! To be safe, follow the manufacturer's recommendations for dilution and store the product out of the reach of pets.

Garage and Basement Substances

Remember, for your pet's (and your children's) safety, keep all garage and basement toxins in tightly closed containers and out of easy-reach. Be sure that you wipe up any traces of the substances after using these products, and dispose of containers, brushes, and rags in properly sealed bags or canisters, in order to avoid spillage and contamination. Frequently check that your automobile is not leaking any toxic substances, as well. Smaller pets can crawl underneath the car and find curious puddles to investigate.

While you are taking safety precautions regarding storage and use, also remember that disposal of cleaning products can be a problem. Americans pour more than 32 million pounds of household cleaning products down the drain every day. Don't forget that these substances contaminate the water systems. If they are not properly filtered out, the toxins invade the drinking water. To avoid further danger to your pet, your family, and your environment, consider purchasing natural products, which avoid both immediate and long-term damage.

Keeping your house clean does not have to harm your pet's health. Natural cleaners and deodorizers worked for great-grandma and they can work for you, too. One of the things you probably love most about your pet is his or her adorable, wide-eyed curiosity. Don't let this inquisitiveness get your animal into a dangerous, painful, possibly fatal situation. Wipe up spills, keep cleaning product containers sealed and out of reach, and allow your pet into a recently-cleaned area only after fumes have dissipated and surfaces have dried.

4.
Lead–
A Lethal Substance

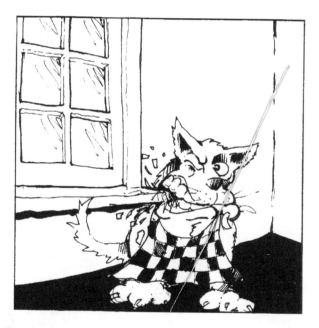

In its original state, lead is an ore in the earth's crust. Because it is durable, resists corrosion, and has a low melting point, lead is indispensable to many industries. Unfortunately, it is also poisonous. Lead paint has been a primary source of lead poisoning over the years. However, due to its ban in 1978, lead paint is now mostly a concern only for those living in older houses. But lead in piping and in faucets continues to cause health problems in many homes and buildings, as it contaminates the tap water. In general, animals are highly susceptible to lead poisoning because of their small size. Symptoms appear in pets before they appear in human children and adults.

The Problem

Lead poisoning is a long-term, serious problem that affects pets and people. In *Everyday Cancer Risks and How to Avoid Them: Effective Ways to Lower Your Odds of Getting Cancer,* Mary Kerney Levenstein explains that when lead enters the body, it first permeates the bloodstream and then travels to the bones and organs. The lead can remain in body tissues for many, many years, continually seeping back into the blood system. It is carried to all parts of the body and results in damage at the cellular level.

A veterinarian can test for lead levels in your pet's bloodstream through a blood test. Often, veterinarians suspect lead poisoning after the pet owner discloses that the animal was chewing on windowsills or that their home

recently has been renovated. But pets can be affected just by breathing lead dust, or they can ingest lead through contaminated drinking water. Young animals are particularly susceptible to lead poisoning, as are young children. The body cannot tell the difference between lead and calcium, and so it 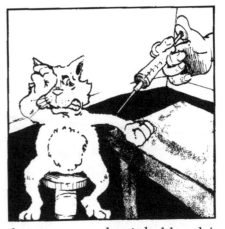 stores lead in the bones in the same way that it holds calcium. This will lead to problems such as neurological symptoms, kidney and reproductive disorders, blindness, and death. Young animals' bodies absorb up to 90 percent of the lead to which they are exposed, whereas adult animals' bodies absorb 10 percent.

Dogs are affected by lead poisoning in much greater numbers than cats, due to the fact that they frequently chew

Symptoms of Lead Poisoning

The symptoms of lead poisoning vary according to the type of animal. Dogs are afflicted with the following symptoms:

- Aimless running
- Anorexia
- Blindness
- Chomping of jaws
- Colic
- Convulsions
- Diarrhea
- Indiscriminate biting
- Kidney problems
- Reproductive disorders
- Restlessness
- Vomiting
- Whining and growling

Lead poisoning causes cats to suffer with:

- Convulsions
- Gastric upset
- Hysteria
- Kidney problems
- Neurological symptoms
- Reproductive disorders

Birds who have been poisoned by lead exhibit:

- Muscle spasms
- Nervous system dysfunction

Lead poisoning may be difficult to detect because, often, the symptoms mimic those of behavioral problems. In fact, dogs are sometimes wrongly diagnosed with canine distemper because the indications are so similar. Identification and treatment is best left to a veterinarian, who will determine the proper *chelation therapy*—a procedure whereby a substance is introduced that binds with another substance (in this case, lead) and is excreted. Under this treatment, animals often improve in twenty-four to forty-eight hours.

wood coated with lead paint. Young dogs—puppies between two and eight months of age—are most affected because they are teething and, therefore, chew almost anything. However, lead poisoning from contaminated drinking water harms pets of *all* ages and species.

Lead Paint

A major source of lead poisoning over the years has been lead paint, which the Consumer Product Safety Commission finally banned in 1978. It took over twenty years for the ban to be passed. In the meantime, measures were taken to reduce the amount of lead used; paint produced after the 1940s reportedly has lower concentrations of lead than older paint.

In 1993, the Environmental Protection Agency estimated that two-thirds of the homes in the United States built before 1940 are contaminated with lead paint (containing up to 50 percent lead). Of the houses erected between 1940 and 1960, one-third have lead paint, and of those constructed since 1960, less than one-third. It is estimated that about 3 million tons of lead remain in 57 million occupied private houses that were built before 1980. Your house could be one of those homes.

Lead paint is typically found in houses built before 1950, on the kitchen and bathroom walls and on doors, windows, shutters, ceilings, railings, stairs, and other forms of woodwork. Most of the toxic surfaces have been painted over. As long as these painted areas are maintained and your animal does not chew the surface, risk of poisoning is low. But do not allow yourself to rely on a false sense of security. If the paint has deteriorated—if it is chipping and flaking— the pulverized lead dust releases into the air. The repeated opening and closing of windows can cause further chipping and, thus, more lead dust. Pets may inhale and walk in this dust, resulting in lead poisoning.

If you are carrying out home renovations and attacking lead-based paint, vacuuming is not enough of a clean-up measure. There are professional ways to rid the environment of the hazard. In painting over lead paint, be careful not to scrape or sand unless you take proper precautions. Lead chips and lead dust can harm your pet, and the residue remains in the air and in floor-cracks for a long time after the renovations are complete. For proper lead paint treatment, read the "Solutions" section of this chapter and contact your local health department or a lead remediation contractor.

Lead-Containing Water and Plumbing Systems

In *Home Magazine*'s "Home Ecology" (April, 1992), D. M. Vandervort reports that the water in as many as 20 percent of American households contains elevated lead levels. This water is contaminated by lead-containing plumbing: lead service pipes, lead water supply pipes, lead-containing faucets, and lead solder. In addition, cisterns continue to be used in some areas to store water or to act as part of rainwater collection systems. Some of these cisterns are constructed with lead liners and/or contain lead solder from construction and repairs. If the water has a relatively low pH, it can dissolve lead from the cistern and cause it to leach into the water. Lead lurks in many public water systems, as old lead pipes carry the water from reservoirs or water facilities to individual homes.

There is no question that lead-pipe plumbing systems are dangerous. Furthermore, systems with copper pipes may contain lead solder. The solder reacts with the copper, creating galvanic corrosion between the two metals and releasing large amounts of lead into the water. Pets that drink this contaminated water can be seriously affected. In 1988, amendments to the Safe Drinking Water Act reduced the acceptable maximum amount of lead in water-pipe solder to 2 percent. Though steps are going in the right direction, the presence of lead is still a concern.

Many faucets contain lead; the inside surfaces of most faucets include, among other materials, lead-containing brass fittings, and some faucets are constructed with lead alloys. It is estimated that one-sixth (approximately 17 percent) of the nation's homes have faucets leaking high

Lead Alert

In 1993, the Environmental Protection Agency estimated that as many as 30 million people served by 819 relatively large public water systems could be drinking water containing unsafe levels of lead. In order to alert you to the hazard of lead in your drinking water, here are several of the U.S. water systems with the highest lead levels:

- Charleston, South Carolina
- Columbia, South Carolina
- Utica, New York
- Yonkers, New York
- Camp Lejeune, North Carolina

Several of the *largest* U.S. water systems that are contaminated with high lead levels are:

- New York, New York
- Philadelphia, Pennsylvania
- Detroit, Michigan
- Washington, District of Columbia
- Boston, Massachusetts
- San Francisco, California

amounts of lead, and newer faucets seem to have the highest concentrations.

Hard water contains considerable amounts of calcium and magnesium that are not properly absorbed and used by the body. However, hard water does tend to form a scale—a build-up of mineral deposits—along the piping, thus creating a protective barrier from contaminants, including lead. *Soft water*—water without calcium and magnesium—is either natural to a location or induced through the use of "water softeners." Unfortunately, it tends to dissolve the lining of pipes, especially when the water is artificially softened, and causes the scale to disappear. Therefore, lead and other toxins leach into the water. When your pet takes a drink from the water dish, lead enters his or her body. To make matters worse, some ceramic water bowls contain lead, heightening the chances of toxic ingestion.

Other Sources of Lead

Sometimes sources that are not commonly suspected are responsible for lead poisoning. Certain driveways are treated with ash that comes from lead smelters. Cats who lay on these driveways can be poisoned if they lick the ash off their fur. It has been reported that a cat got lead poisoning by sitting on a windowsill next to an area that contained a large amount of automobile fumes; at that time, lead was still an ingredient in gasoline. Birds who peck at lead ceramics, lead putty, lead paint on their cages, and lead curtain weights are at risk of being poisoned. Yet, an encouraging observation has been made that guinea pigs whose cages are often lined with newspapers have a high tolerance to the lead found in the ink on the papers; there are no recorded instances of adverse reactions. Further sources of lead include crystal, pottery, older food storage cans, concrete, soil, dust, and toys that are decorated with lead paint.

The Solution

Detection is the first step in resolving concerns about lead poisoning. You do not have to do guess-work; there are competent tests available. Then, you can prevent further harm from occurring by removing lead at its source or by bolstering your environment with safety measures.

Lead Paint

If your surfaces have been painted before 1978, chances are that lead-based paint was used. But regardless of when the most recent painting job occurred, for the health of your pet and your family, check your house. The process of detecting lead in your home is not difficult or lengthy. An older home should be tested with a kit specifically designed for lead paint. Hardware stores carry easy-to-use kits that do the job well. They involve a simple method of evaluating a surface area; the tip of the tester turns pink or red if lead is present. There are also testers that indicate lead in dishes, on toys, in soil, etc., in addition to lead in wall and surface paint. If lead paint is found, you should hire a professional lead remediation company. The service will determine the extent of the contaminated area through laboratory testing of samples taken at specified distances, or through an x-ray fluorescence analyzer (XRF) test on the walls. The XRF test detects the presence of lead on the subsurface with the use of a machine. These tests will reveal whether it is necessary to do a complete renovation or simply to remodel certain areas.

Where extensive areas of lead paint are found, the safest solution is to replace the painted surface. This is best done by a licensed contractor, who will take the proper precautions to contain any dust that may be released into the air. This dust can be extremely hazardous if inhaled by you, your children, or your pet. Licensed remediation contractors encapsulate the area in a plastic bubble, use dampening substances to restrict the dust, and remove the toxic material with water vacuums. For cases of lead in soil, they apply exterior soil containment methods. It is advised that you move out of the home during renovations, in order to avoid contact with the lead dust. This includes taking your pets with you! For a list of approved lead-removal contractors, contact your state health office. *Never* attempt removal yourself.

In order to protect your pet from lead paint that is covered and in good condition, routinely clean the floors, windowsills, baseboards, and other surfaces with either a trisodium phosphate cleaner or phosphate-free *LFA-11*—a detergent specifically developed for lead-contaminated dust removal. As with the use of all chemicals, keep pets away until the surfaces are dry and the fumes have dissipated. Treat wood surfaces with a pet repellent to prevent your animal from chewing them; the repellent will smell repulsive to your pet. For paint that is chipping, tape the area until you can have the paint removed, thus preventing further deterioration. If the area spans across walls, cover it with new paint, wallpaper, or paneling. In general, before you sand and do any renovations, determine the constitution of the old paint.

Try to keep your house as free as possible from lead dust. Replace carpets if lead dust is suspected, as there is *no* completely safe way to remove lead dust from these floor coverings. If you clean the carpets with a vacuum, the dust can get tossed into the air and inhaled, or land on tables, dishes, and other objects.

Although lead paint is not used in more recently built houses, pets can still develop illnesses by ingesting dust from other types of commercial chemical-based paints. A good rule of thumb is to keep animals away from all work areas during renovation, and to use proper clean-up methods.

Lead-Containing Water and Plumbing Systems

The first step in protecting your family and your pet from lead poisoning caused by contaminated water is to purchase a home lead-in-water test kit, which will give you an indication of whether further professional analysis is necessary. These tests are designed for easy use. If water tests reveal the presence of lead, do not give your animal companion water from the tap. Instead, give your pet bottled water or install a water filtration system. For situations in which you *must* use tap water, let the faucet run for two minutes prior to filling the dish. This will help to flush out the system and dispose of water that has accumulated lead while standing in the pipes.

Where the piping is the problem, it is best to replace lead plumbing. If this solution is not feasible, or if lead is coming from your water supply lines, the only solution is to use point-of-use or whole-house filtration. Point-of-use filters remedy the situation for an individual faucet, while whole-house filtration attends to the lead problem at the main water pipe. Common effective methods are carbon fil-tration, distillation, and reverse osmosis. (For information on how these filtering systems work, see "City Water," page 85.) Granulated active carbon (GAC) filters, found in many inexpensive commercial point-of-use filters, may not suffi-ciently remove lead if used by themselves. When purchasing a filtration system, you should make sure that the manufac-turer *guarantees* lead removal.

Other Sources of Lead

As previously discussed, kits that rely on surface-testing are available and easy-to-use. Simply touch the test to the toy, pot-tery, etc., and observe the color change. Avoid the use of any pet dishes containing lead, and never buy food in cans made with lead solder. Look for the term "lead-free" on the can.

If soil is suspected or found to be contaminated, fence off that area and plant grass to keep the dust down. Animals who have been exposed to lead-contaminated soil should have their fur and paws washed before they enter the house.

Lead is a highly toxic substance for both pets and people. Any family whose pet is diagnosed with lead poisoning should have their children tested immediately. Puppies give clues as to the impending lead poisoning of young children. They live and eat in the same environment, and develop identifiable signs of lead poisoning long before symptoms are obvious in children.

Even if your bird, cat, or dog does not show symptoms of lead poisoning, take detection measures if your house fits the criteria for possibly having lead paint. Do not wait for severe signs of poisoning to occur, for by then, too much suf-fering already will have taken place.

5.
Plants That Poison

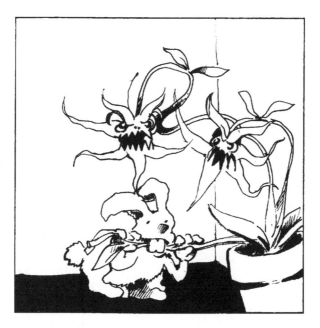

Animals tend to consume plants as a natural way to improve their health. For example, cats normally eat grass for nutrition, as well as to induce vomiting for the removal of hairballs. But there are many cases in which pets accidentally ingest toxins from poisonous plants, resulting in sickness. Common indoor and outdoor plants can cause illness and, in extreme cases, death. Cats may scratch plants and become infected when grooming their claws. Dogs may randomly chew or eat plants that emit intriguing scents. Therefore, it is important to be familiar with the types of plants in your area and to keep the toxic ones out of your pet's paths.

The Problem

Catnip is an example of a relatively harmless plant that simply intoxicates the kitty. But other common house and yard plants have lethal effects on our animal friends. The best way to prevent plant poisoning is to familiarize yourself with common dangerous plants, and to either remove them from the premises or carefully monitor your pet's favorite spots.

Plants that are naturally nontoxic to animals can still make your pet sick if the vegetation has been sprayed with pesticides or fertilizers. Also, if toxins are applied to an already-poisonous plant, clinical signs of illness from the plant itself may be masked or altered. Finally, if your animal companion has particular sensitivities, even plants that are nontoxic to the general animal population and plants that are not sprayed with chemicals might cause stomach upset in your pet.

Outdoor pets are especially at risk of plant poisoning. There is little you can do to monitor your neighbor's yard or the woods behind your house. However, you have control over your indoor plants and those on your own property. If you suspect that your pet is hungrily "eyeing" the plants, confirm that they are nontoxic.

Irritating plants commonly cause skin rashes—allergic dermatitis—in both pets and humans. If your animal develops a skin condition, trace his or her "haunts" to determine if a toxic plant may be causing the problem. You might not be able to identify harmful plants yourself, but observe the vegetation and report anything that you find suspicious or unfamiliar to the veterinarian. As with all symptomatic conditions, the veterinarian will be able to offer better treatment if he or she knows the entire story.

Symptoms of Plant Poisoning

While specific symptoms of plant poisoning depend on the type of toxic plant that is ingested, there are some general indications of which you should be aware. For dogs and cats, these include:

- Breathing difficulties
- Convulsions
- Excessive salivation
- Gastroenteritis
- Irritation of mouth and lips
- Skin rashes
- Stomach upset
- Swallowing difficulties
- Vomiting
- Watery eyes and nose

Birds instinctively know which seeds to avoid, so it is unlikely that they will be poisoned by toxic plants. In addition, caged birds' diets are very controllable and, thus, poisoning is not generally a threat. However, wild birds *will* be harmed by the pesticides applied to plants from which they derive their seeds, in which cases they will experience the following symptoms:

- Drooping wings
- Erratic flight
- Head tremors
- Hormonal changes
- Listlessness
- Paralysis
- Regurgitation
- Reproductive disorders
- Respiratory stress and possibly failure
- Ruffled feathers
- Shortness of breath
- Side-to-side head movements
- Vomiting

Indoor Plants

Decorative house plants can be as poisonous as they are pretty. Dieffenbachia inflames the mouth and lips of some dogs, cats, and birds. It may also interfere with breathing and swallowing. Philodendron has been known to cause irritation of the mucous membranes and excessive salivation in cats. Daffodils and Indian rubber plants are also toxic.

Dried flower arrangements are a beautiful addition to a home's decor, but often contain toxic plants. Hydrangea and bittersweet have been known to provoke gastroenteritis. Furthermore, the ingestion of bittersweet can result in unconsciousness.

Plants are a common form of holiday decoration. While you are preparing festive arrangements, know which species are dangerous to your pet. Mistletoe, if eaten, can be lethal to a dog. Poinsettias may cause vomiting and even death to any household pet. Even Christmas tree needles and the water from the base of the tree can provoke gastrointestinal distress. Easter lilies are poisonous to cats.

Outdoor Plants

Common yard plants such as laurel, rhododendrons, and azaleas may inflict your pet with watery eyes, a runny nose, vomiting, convulsions, and, in the case of laurel, death. Daphne, lantanas, holly, and wormwood are also harmful shrubs. Garden flowers to be wary of include delphiniums, foxglove, monkshood, irises, lilies of the valley, amaryllis, morning glories, and daffodils. Easter lilies and tiger lilies are especially toxic for cats. Bulbs are a favorite treat of dogs who do a lot of digging, so take necessary precaution. The bulbs of daffodils, narcissus, and jonquils trigger severe gastroenteritis. Hyacinth bulbs cause trembling and convulsions.

Among the trees that bear poisonous seeds, blossoms, and/or leaves, etc., are oak; peach; cherry; elderberry; black locust; apple; and oleander. Even some vegetable plants harm pets, including avocado leaves and unripe stems; rhubarb leaves; spinach leaves; and tomato vines, stems, and leaves. Dangerous wild plants include Jack-in-the-pulpit; moonseed; May apple; Dutchman's breeches; water hemlock; mushrooms;

buttercup; nightshade; poison hemlock; jimsonweed; pigweed; locoweed; lupine; heliotrope; poison ivy; and poison oak.

The Solution

If you are in a panic because you think your pet has been poisoned and you are unable to get to a veterinarian immediately, there is a group that can provide you with emergency service—the ASPCA's National Animal Poison Control Center. It is the first animal-oriented poison center in the United States. The center's phones are answered by licensed veterinarians and board certified veterinary toxicologists. Do not call your local human poison control center, as they are not well-versed in treatments for pets. The National Animal Poison Control Center has extensive experience with over 250,000 cases involving plants, pesticides, drugs, metals, and other toxic exposures that have harmed pets and food-producing animals. There is a charge for consultation. For telephone numbers and cost information, please see the Information Resources list, page 115.

The National Animal Poison Control Center also publishes a large booklet on the most common plants that cause poisoning, and explains associated problems and hazards. The price of the packet is $10. To receive this publication or for further information on their services, write to the address given in the Information Resources list.

Indoor Plants

The solution to the problem of indoor plant poisoning is to arrange your decor carefully. Where possible, avoid the presence of toxic plants. Even if a plant is on a high shelf or tucked far back on a window sill, leaves and blossoms can still fall onto the carpet, and cats, especially, can find ways to wiggle into tight, unlikely spots. If you are set on keeping certain "risky" plants, be sure to perch them out of your pet's reach.

Around the holidays, refamiliarize yourself with the toxicity of seasonal plants and either avoid them or place the plants in a secure area, away from your pet. If you purchase real Christmas trees and mistletoe, try to keep your animal in the safer rooms of the house and be on careful watch.

Outdoor Plants

Again, protecting your pet from dangerous plants first involves familiarizing yourself with which species are harmful. Then, either fence off areas where toxic plants are found, or remove the plants entirely. If you have a dog who likes to dig, avoid daffodils, narcissus, jonquils, and hyacinth bulbs, or put them in a location where the dog can't get to them.

Some pet owners allow their animals to roam in unrestricted areas. This is dangerous for a number of reasons; toxic plant contact is only one of many hazards. However, if your pet does travel around the neighborhood, trace his or her steps and confirm that there is no threat of plant poisoning. You may readily recognize clusters of certain toxic vegetation, such as poison ivy, poisonous mushrooms, and buttercup. But other dangerous plants are more obscure. The plants that have been named in this chapter are pictured in most plant encyclopedias and botanical resource books.

As in any emergency, medical treatment must be sought if you suspect that your pet has been poisoned by a plant. Time is of the essence and poisoning, whether from a plant or another source, should be considered a life or death situation. If a veterinarian cannot be reached immediately, call the poison control center discussed above. Remember, it is difficult to diagnose plant poisoning from other types of illness, so to help the diagnostic process if your animal companion becomes ill, know what plants are in and around your home and the dangers associated with them.

6.
Problematic Pesticides & Toxic Flea Treatments

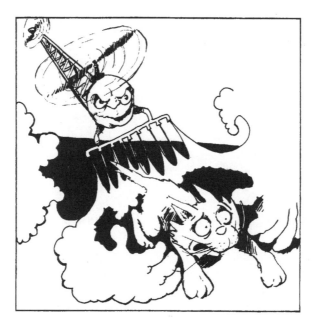

M̲ost of us have an aversion to insects and will do almost anything to rid our homes and yards of them, whether the bugs are harmful or not. But the costs could be outweighing the benefits. The chemicals that are used in extermination can have severely detrimental effects on both pet and human health. Pesticides that eliminate insects (especially fleas, ticks, and termites) and

Symptoms of Pesticide and Chemical Flea Treatment Poisoning

The chemicals in pesticides and most commercial flea repellents are fat-soluble and are stored in the fatty tissues of the body, primarily in the liver, and in the nervous system. As these chemicals accumulate over time, they negatively affect nerves, hormones, and immunity. The actual symptoms that an animal exhibits depend on the type of toxic substance involved. However, there are some general symptoms for which you should watch. Dogs and cats demonstrate the following:

- Anorexia
- Cancer
- Colic
- Convulsions
- Deformity of sexual organs
- Depression
- Diarrhea
- Foaming at the mouth
- Gastroenteritis
- Increased respiratory rate
- Infertility
- Irritability
- Nausea
- Nervousness
- Seizures
- Stiffness
- Vomiting
- Weakness

In birds, symptoms of pesticide poisoning include:

- Drooping wings
- Erratic flight
- Head tremors
- Hormonal changes
- Listlessness
- Paralysis
- Regurgitation
- Reproductive disorders
- Respiratory stress and possibly failure
- Ruffled feathers
- Shortness of breath
- Side-to-side head movements
- Vomiting

rodents, as well as weeds and fungi, are sold in many forms: sprays, liquids, balls, sticks, powders, crystals, and foggers.

According to the Environmental Protection Agency, there are more than 34,000 pesticides in use in the United States, and these substances are the second highest cause of household poisonings in humans. The statistics may be even higher for dogs and cats, considering that many pets indiscriminately ingest toxic substances by licking up chemical residue or grooming it off their fur.

The Problem

Insecticides can disrupt the biological processes of an animal's body, resulting in effects that include the feminizing of male animals and the disrupting of their ability to reproduce. According to *Food and Water Newsletter* (Marshfield, Vermont), a Florida study that took place from 1985 to 1990 reported that 67 percent of male panthers were born with at least one undescended testicle, causing infertility. Researchers found that these animals had twice as much estrogen in their bodies as testosterone. Lab analysis pointed to estrogenic chemicals, primarily pesticides, as the cause of these hormonal problems. The same study revealed that female seagulls under observation were found to be sharing nests with other females and were not interested in mating. Situations like these are critical in the wild, as they worsen the state of endangered species.

Although our cats, dogs, and birds are not in danger of extinction, long-term exposure to pesticides can have other serious consequences for these animals, including chronic disease. The above-mentioned study proves that pesticides and chemical flea treatments have highly toxic properties that disturb the proper functioning of the body.

Agricultural Sprays

The spraying of agricultural chemicals can affect any animal caught in the line of fire—in the immediate area, as well as those downwind of the spraying. Not only do animals eat food sprayed with pesticides, but they also ingest toxins by breathing air in recently sprayed areas and by grooming their contaminated fur. Dogs are more susceptible to contamination through inhalation of chemicals, whereas cats more often ingest toxins because they lick their coats. Furthermore, if the agricultural pesticides leach into the water supply, animals may be poisoned simply by drinking the water. Chlordane, DDT, and lindane are just a few of the agricultural sprays that are potential killers. They remain in the air and on the ground for years, and have long-term effects on the body. For example, chlordane has a half-life—the length of time that it takes for half of the given amount to be processed (metabolized or eliminated) by the biological functions of an organism—of fifty years. In 1980, the EPA banned this substance from termite pesticides. DDE, a byproduct of DDT, has been found in the tumors of some breast cancer patients. It is believed that, years prior, these women ingested DDT through contaminated food. Female pets are at risk, as well.

Animals that are poisoned by pesticides from agricultural sprays may exhibit foaming at the mouth, irritability, increased respiratory rate, and even seizures. If proper treatment is not administered immediately, the animal can die. Seek advice from your veterinarian or a poison control center as soon as possible.

Common Household Pesticides

The toxic effects of household pesticides should not be underestimated. Insecticides containing chlorinated hydrocarbons are dangerous, especially to birds. Within forty-eight hours of exposure to these chemicals, birds can exhibit the symptoms listed on page 62, and can even die while airborne and in erratic flight.

Strychnine, used in many pesticides, is especially lethal for dogs and cats. Signs of poisoning, such as apprehension and stiffness, can appear within several minutes of ingestion. Convulsions develop as the poison spreads throughout the body. Eventually, respiratory arrest causes death. In their article, "Clinical Toxicities of Cats," veterinarians Clarke

Atkins and Roger Johnson describe a case of strychnine poisoning in a dog who had remained indoors for over twelve hours. It was discovered that the family cat had found a strychnine-laced meatball, brought it into the house, and then decided it was not edible. Unfortunately, the dog did not share the same instinct and ate part of the meatball. As a result, the dog was poisoned. Birds can also become casualties of strychnine poisoning, especially if they eat strychnine-laced seed that is prepared as mouse poison. Symptoms include paralysis and respiratory failure.

Arsenic, which is used in insecticides, herbicides, ant poisons, snail bait, paints, and some drugs, can cause acute poisoning, triggering the following symptoms: severe gastroenteritis; depression; colic; anorexia; extreme weakness; and death. Cats and small dogs exhibit these symptoms within thirty minutes of ingesting large doses, and can die within seven hours. Large dogs experience effects that are less severe, but certainly detrimental. Birds react with ruffled feathers, drooping wings, anorexia, and regurgitation.

Keep in mind that one reason why household pets are affected by toxins more often than humans is because of their size. An amount of toxin that is considered small and therefore "safe" for humans is proportionally larger for your animal companion. Therefore, be sure to understand the toxic properties of extermination substances. Avoid putting your special animal friend at great risk of suffering.

Flea Treatments

Everyone hates fleas and will go to great lengths to keep them away. In fact, it is considered a necessary service to keep pets as free of fleas as possible. Unfortunately, as is the case with other pest control methods, many of the substances that are marketed as beneficial to pets actually can bring serious harm to them.

Pyrethrum is a nontoxic insecticide made from chrysanthemum flowers and used as a flea repellent. It is considered safe in its natural state; reactions usually are limited to increased salivation because of pyrethrum's bitter taste, although it can be harmful to frogs and reptiles. However, many pyrethrum products contain chemical additives that are dangerous for dogs and cats, causing such symptoms as vomiting, diarrhea, mild tremors, hyperexcitability, severe hypersalivation, depression, and seizures. These symptoms usually last for up to three days, unless the animal is re-exposed. Read labels carefully and use only natural pyrethrum powders.

One popular ingredient in insect repellents for humans is *diethyl toluamide* (DEET). It is estimated that, annually, 22 percent of the general population in the United States is exposed to DEET-based products, especially mosquito repellents. This substance can also be found in some flea repellents. Certain symptoms related to nervous disorders can arise with repeated use of DEET on pets. Furthermore, in 1990, the Washington Toxic Coalition (Dorman, District of Columbia) reported that cats have died from repeated fleabaths containing DEET. Cats and dogs develop tremors, vomiting, excitation, and seizures. This substance has been proven to penetrate the skin of guinea pigs within six hours and may cause problems with the central nervous system. Human children can also be affected, exhibiting signs of lethargy, behavioral changes, abnormal movements, seizures, and coma, as well as chemical burns to sensitive skin. It is safest to choose a less toxic alternative.

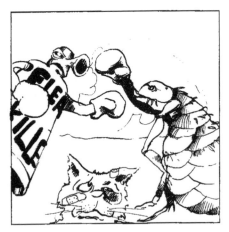

Chemical flea collars pose a threat to small animals. Some contain *DDVP*, which is supposedly nontoxic for dogs, but sensitive animals can suffer excessive salivation, diarrhea, and respiratory difficulties due to this substance. The constant inhalation of DDVP fumes can cause permanent damage to internal organs. And remember, as the size of the animal decreases, the risk of toxic effects increases. Flea collars that include *dichlorvos* among their ingredients may cause contact dermatitis in some pets. In addition, commercial flea collars use chemicals that *claim* to kill the pests, but fleas often hop over the collars and inhabit the pet's face. Therefore, you may be exposing your pet to harmful chemicals that don't even serve their purpose! Most chemical flea collars come with warnings about their toxicity, but the whole story isn't told: "dust from this collar is harmful if swallowed and may cause eye problems"; "if not removed from pets during baths, make sure shampoo contaminated with collar dust does not get into the eyes"; "follow disposal directions properly."

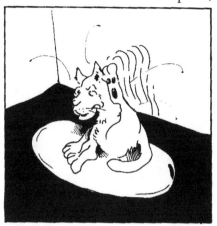

Foggers or "bombs" are often used to get rid of fleas that have infested the home. Warnings on these products indicate that the fumes are dangerous and that the mist, which settles over the area, is harmful when inhaled or when absorbed through the skin; food and cooking surfaces should be covered; vehicles should be removed from garages; and aquariums and plants should be protected prior to use. Instructions state that people and pets should vacate the home during use, but may return after the fumes have dissipated. However, the chemicals used in flea bombs have half-lives of more than fifty years. Therefore, if foggers are employed, you will be living with toxins inside your home, and so will the next owner of the house. Active ingredients in foggers include DDVP, propoxur, diazinon, and carbaryl, all of which are nerve poisons to both pets and humans. Their residues remain in furnishings, carpets, drapes, and wood. And unfortunately, despite this assault on your house, the fleas don't stay away! Repeated "bombings" are necessary, increasing the chance for sickness each time.

Many people develop allergies after fumigation, some of which last for as long as the family lives in the house. The harmful substances cannot be removed unless the house is gutted, and, ultimately, it may be more feasible to move. Since pets spend a lot of time indoors, they may be developing allergic reactions. In addition, respiration problems and even cancer are suspected consequences.

Garden and Lawn Chemicals

Many gardeners believe that the key to growing a successful crop of vegetables or a beautiful flower garden is to keep these areas free from insects and weeds. Homeowners tend to feel this way about their lawns and shrubs, as well. To accomplish these goals, people often use large amounts of potentially toxic chemicals without considering the effects that these substances may have on pets and other animals.

In her book titled *Nontoxic, Natural and Earthwise*, Debra Lynn Dadd reveals that Americans use approximately 300 million pounds of (indoor and outdoor) pesticides per year; 91 percent of American households take part in this problem. The majority of these chemicals are long-lasting and insoluble in water, and can poison your pet.

Rotenone is derived from the derris plant and applied as a garden and shrub pesticide. It is described as semi-toxic; studies have proven that, if ingested by cats, rotenone may cause nausea, vomiting, and future liver damage. Sabadilla, which comes from the seeds of a South American lily and also is used in gardens and on shrubs, is considered less toxic than many other pesticides, but it is harmful to bees and humans who come in direct contact with it. Considering this fact, how harmless can it be for pets to walk or roll in plants that are treated with this substance? Sometimes nicotine is applied to plants because it, too, is considered less poisonous than other pesticides, but dogs, cats, birds, and fish can die if they eat it. Remember, an insecticide that is labeled "nontoxic" is not necessarily safe for your pet.

Cats and dogs are not immune to insect sprays. They can be affected not only through ingestion of contaminated food, but from direct contact with the pesticide, as well. Any animal rummaging around in the garden, whether it is your dog, a rabbit, or a raccoon, may become covered in spray residue. This can cause skin disorders and can affect the internal organs, as animals are likely to ingest the toxins when they groom their fur.

Lawn fertilizers and weed and insect killers often contain the following hazardous chemicals: 2,4,D; banvel; benomyl; chloropyrifos; daconil; and diazinon. The most potent and widely used weed-killer is 2,4,D; it has been proven to cause depression, loss of memory, paranoia, irritability, and cancer. Verification of many of these symptoms came from animal studies, so our pets suffer the same symptoms and consequences as we do. A study reported in the *Journal of the National Cancer Institute* found that dogs who were exposed to repeated applications of 2,4,D were twice as likely to get malignant lymphoma as dogs who were not exposed. Toxic weed killers should never be used by pet owners whose animals go outside and come into contact with the contaminated areas.

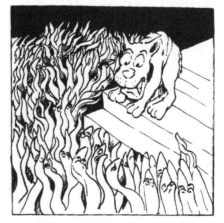

Many people lovingly treat the wild birds as pets and kindly feed them during the winter season. It is important to continue concern for these creatures and not to poison them in the warmer months by spraying flowers, fruits, and vegetables with pesticides. Birds can also be harmed by airborne contaminants from sprays.

Rat Poison

Rodent bait is not only poisonous to rats; it is also hazardous to your animal companion. In fact, some pet-haters will purposely put this toxin out as a poison against neighborhood dogs and cats. Rat poison causes symptoms such as nervousness, restlessness, muscle rigidity, convulsions, profuse salivation, nausea, and diarrhea. If you notice any of these symptoms in your pet, contact a veterinarian immediately.

The Solution ██████████████████

Fortunately, it is not necessary to rely on harsh, potentially dangerous chemicals to remove pests from your home, your garden, and your pet's fur. There are many simple, natural solutions to these problems.

Agricultural Sprays

After studies showed that the chemical spraying of crops had terrible long-term effects on the population, such as an increase in cancer cases, several chemicals were banned. Among these is *DDT*, which is suspected as being responsible for a rise in breast cancer. More and more farmers are turning to organic (non-chemical) methods not necessarily because they are purists, but because pesticides don't work anymore. Pests have developed such a strong resistance to pesticides that the quantity of toxins needed for effective crop protection costs more than the average farmer can afford. Integrated Pest Management (IPM) is a methodology in which insects are controlled through biological and other means that are environmentally friendly, for the most part. It employs a combination of organic and chemical remedies, and aims to reduce the amount of chemical ingredients until only the natural substances are used. IPM applies as many nontoxic remedies as possible, such as a botanical insecticide, extracted from the seeds of the neem tree, that repels armyworms, aphids, and Japanese beetles. Horticultural oils, such as *Sunspray Oil*, that smother insects instead of poisoning them are also becoming more popular. *Gardens Alive* is one of the many catalog sources that lists these types of products. (See the Information Resources list, page 115, for more information.)

Common Household Pesticides

It is destructive, but nonetheless easy, to rely on the well-advertised, chemically charged insecticide sprays that are available in stores. However, natural remedies are healthier and also readily available. We recommend *Bugs Off*, an all-natural spray that is manufactured by Nature's Path. Also, ants and roaches are repelled by lemongrass and by borates, which effectively eliminate these pests for up to a year or more. Tea tree oil and eucalyptus oil are considered insect repellents, but should only be used in diluted form; concentrated amounts of these substances may cause near-fatal poisonings in pets and children. The *heatwave system* is a safe way to get rid of termites; this method "cooks" wood to temperatures of 130° F and kills the insects. Contact a professional exterminator for more information.

If you are enjoying an evening on the back porch, use rosemary, bay leaves, or citronella to keep bugs away. Mosquito problems in your yard can be remedied with the use of citronella-based repellents found in many health food stores. Also, install bird houses to attract purple martins, or bat houses to encourage bat colonies; both will devastate mosquito populations. Bats, especially, are beneficial creatures and should not be treated as predators.

Flea Treatments

With all of the worries that come along with using chemical-containing shampoos, dips, and flea collars, it is best to choose only natural, nontoxic flea remedies. There are safe products that use pennyroyal, eucalyptus, cedar, and citronella. Some animals will exhibit a salivation reaction to certain herbs and may not be able to wear them. As an alternative, sprinkle nutritional yeast—not brewers yeast, which can cause skin problems, allergies, and vomiting—in your pet's food once a day, and you will be pleasantly surprised to see no more fleas! Apparently, the ingredients in yeast cause a certain skin odor that makes the animal unappetizing to fleas and ticks. You can also use garlic or sulfur, both of which cause a reaction that emits hydrogen sulfide on the surface of the pet's skin. Wakunaga of America, Ltd. makes a liquid garlic extract called *Kyolic,* which is easy to administer orally. Sulfur is a byproduct of mineral supplements; it is not put in food or applied topically. Amidst all of these remedies, do not forget that flea combs and nontoxic flea sprays can tackle the problem when you groom your pet, if you have the time.

If fleas invade your animal companion, they may also invade your home. Instead of using foggers or "bombs," bake the fleas out! This method should be done by a professional exterminator. It involves removing all living things from your home and turning on the heat as high as it will go. After approximately one day, the fleas will be dead. Another solution is found in carpet and bedding sprays that contain citronella, eucalyptus, and lemongrass oils. These do a much better job than chemical foggers and sprays, and generally do not make pets or people sick. However, beware of solutions containing undiluted forms of citrus extracts, as they can be harmful to animals, especially cats. (See page 43 for more information on undiluted citrus oils.) Furthermore, if you select a flea repellent that uses pyrethrum, remember that only *natural* pyrethrum products are safe. Some flea powders contain both pyrethrum and chemical additives, which combine to form a toxic substance. Oil from the pennyroyal plant is an effective flea treatment, but should not be used on pregnant animals. Finally, there are "flea birth-control hormones"—methoprene and fenoxycarb—that are available through veterinarians. These substances prevent flea eggs and larvae from maturing into adults and are available in sprays and flea collars.

Outdoors, you may try sprinkling flea-eating nematodes—plant-like worms that will not harm your pet—in areas where your animal lies down. Nematodes are available through catalogs such as *Gardens Alive* and in organic garden stores. They need moisture to survive, so once you spread them, keep the area damp.

Garden and Lawn Chemicals

A healthy alternative to the chemical removal of weeds in the garden and on the lawn is to dig them out by hand. Though it is time-consuming and physically laborious, you will be providing a much safer environment for your pet and your family by avoiding toxic substances. And don't forget the added benefits of exercise and fresh air!

Also consider *companion planting*, a natural method of protecting your yard from destructive insects. For example, certain insects will not eat carrots if they grow next to tomatoes. Thus, planting these two species next to each other will naturally eliminate the threat of certain insect damage to the crop. Also, strong plants are less likely to attract predators. By properly feeding your plants with kelp, compost, and minerals, you can strengthen and protect them. Organic gardeners never use pesticides. There are many helpful books that have been written on organic gardening and companion planting, including Louise Riotte's *Carrots Love Tomatoes*, and Clue Tyler Dennis' and Luke Miller's *If You Like My Apples: A Simple Guide to Biodynamic Gardening*.

Rat Poison

If an animal ingests rat poison, medical attention may not be successful in preventing permanent damage or death. Therefore, the best preventative method is to know your pet's "haunts" and to patrol them often for poisons. If you suspect that your pet has been in contact with rodent bait, contact a veterinarian immediately.

The consuming public has become accustomed to purchasing bottles and cans of chemical remedies. Yet the ingestion and inhalation of pesticide powders, bombs, sprays, etc. expose both pets and people to potentially disastrous conditions. Natural alternatives are far safer and work just as well. If you think about your animal companion and how important he or she is in your life, perhaps it will be easier to break the reliance on harmful pesticides and chemical flea treatments and to start researching alternatives. Pets naturally do things that put them at risk, such as licking their fur and rummaging through substance-treated gardens. They are helplessly exposed to a chemically-treated environment. It is in your power to offer your pet a healthier, happier life through the use of natural pesticide solutions.

7.
Water Contamination Concerns

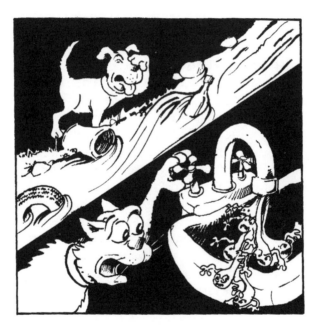

W ater has the ability to dissolve almost all substances with which it comes into contact It carries
dissolved solids—particulates in the water, including dust, dirt, metal, asbestos, and other contaminants—as
suspended matter, as well as bacteria and biologicals, which
include organisms like cryptosporidium. These harmful
substances infest drinking and bathing water and pose

health risks to both you and your animal companion. Your pet relies on you to supply fresh water, but due to the large-scale contamination problems that affect countless regions, you are likely to be offering him or her a liquid containing chlorine, fluoride, nitrates, lead, arsenic, pesticides, and mercury (among other things). While you cannot single-handedly purify the entire water supply, you can remedy the problem within your own home and offer your animal a better quality of life.

The Problem

The polluted water supply is a frightening issue. Health departments often warn the public against consuming mercury-contaminated fish, and they discuss the dangers of eating shellfish that feed near industrial areas. Every now and then, the media spreads awareness of a bacteria in the drinking water that harms entire neighborhoods. Water treatment facilities have been created to help clean the water supply, but many are underfunded and lack the proper equipment to do the job properly. And tainted water is not just an urban problem. Well water can be contaminated with agricultural runoff and industrial ground pollution.

Animals are somewhat resistant to biological contamination; they do not become sick every time they drink from a stream or a muddy puddle. Yet chemical contamination does affect their health and may be creating long-term chronic illness that cannot even be anticipated at present. It is essential that pets drink clean water and maintain a proper mineral balance. Therefore, a responsible pet owner has his or her tap water tested. In some cases, local or state water departments and/or health departments analyze water at no charge. However, since these agencies usually test only for bacteria, not toxic chemicals, the best alternative is to contact a commercial laboratory or state university laboratory and test your tap water through them. If contaminants are found, install a water filter and, if necessary, add the minerals that are absent.

Symptoms Caused by Contaminated Water

Symptoms of contaminated water poisoning in pets will vary, depending on the type of pollutant that is causing the problem. However, there are some general indications for which you should watch. For dogs and cats, these symptoms include:

- Anorexia
- Cancer
- Dental fluorosis (staining of teeth)
- Distemper-like symptoms (in dogs only)
- Eczema
- Gastric upset
- Hormonal changes
- Nausea
- Neurological disorders
- Restlessness
- Skin rash
- Vomiting

Birds who have been affected by contaminated water suffer the following symptoms:

- Cancer
- Hormonal changes
- Neurological disorders
- Restlessness
- Vomiting

City Water

About half of the nation's drinking water comes from ground water aquifers that lie anywhere from 20 to 1,000-feet beneath the earth's surface. The aquifers are porous formations consisting of layers of sand, gravel, or rock. Amidst these layers are areas that allow water to collect above nonporous sheets of bedrock. The subsurface water moves very slowly, sometimes as little as three feet per year. Without sun or oxygen to cleanse it, contamination is a constant threat. Pollutants that leach through the ground can accumulate to dangerous levels in the aquifers. When these water sources are tapped for drinking and bathing use, health hazards become an ugly reality.

Drinking Water Worries

Contaminated water triggers many of the same illnesses in pets as it does in humans. Therefore, although the following statistics refer to humans, we can assume that our pets are being affected in the same ways.

- According to "Preventing Lead Poisoning in Young Children" (October, 1991), published by the Department of Health and Human Services in Atlanta, Georgia, one in six people drink water with excessive amounts of lead in it.

- *Water Technology*'s "News Bulletins" from the June 1994 issue reveals that microbes in tap water may be responsible for one in three cases of gastrointestinal illness.

- The June 1994 issue of *Water Technology* cites an Environmental Protection Agency study reporting that in Ohio's eighty-eight counties, death rates from bladder and stomach cancer were higher where drinking water was taken from rivers and lakes, as compared with where it came from wells.

- In an article from the July 1994 edition of *Water Technology*, the Natural Resources Defense Council claims that more than 350,000 people drink water with arsenic levels above the federal limit. Furthermore, the limit has been criticized as being much too lenient.

Landfills have been known to hold over 200 toxic substances, including numerous chemical compounds. With 16,000 dumps in use in the United States, potentially 8 million people and pets could be affected when those substances leach into ground water. There are about 2.3 million gasoline tanks buried underground, and an estimated 25 percent of these are leaking. Furthermore, many industrial chemical tanks pollute ground water.

Agricultural runoff containing fertilizers, animal manure, and pesticides also taint the water supply. Each year, 25 to 30 million acres of lawns in the United States are fertilized. Suburban landscapers use two-and-a-half times more pesticides per acre than farmers do, and the runoff goes into underground water sources. About 20 percent of all public ground water supplies contain 5 pesticides.

In an effort to remove these pollutants, city water suppliers employ elaborate filtration systems. They also add substances such as chlorine to kill bacteria, and fluoride to "help" our teeth. But these substances can do more harm than good.

Chlorine

Chlorine has been praised as the answer to combating biological pollutants in drinking water and swimming pools. However, the labels on packages of chlorine refer to the substance as a poison and list numerous precautions for its use. If chlorine is strongly effective against unwanted microorganisms, what can it be doing to the cells inside a living body?

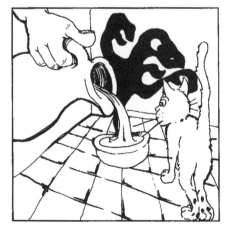

Studies have found it likely that more than 1 person in 10,000 will be inflicted with cancer as a result of water chlorination. Chlorine reacts with other organic (carbon-based) materials and produces hundreds of chemical byproducts called *trihalomethanes* (THMs), several of which cause cancer in animals. Among the THMs are the following known carcinogens: carbon tetrachloride, bis-chloroethane, and chloroform. These toxic substances are turning up in most cities' water supplies.

According to "Clinton Clean Water Plan May Ban Chlorine, EPA Says," in *Water Technology* (June 1994), a United States Public Health Service study researching the effects of chlorinated drinking water on humans linked chlorinated water to premature births, low birth weights, and increased risk of bladder and rectal cancer. These studies were conducted with total trihalomethane levels of 80 parts per billion (ppb). The federal maximum is 100 ppb. There is no reason to believe that pets' bodies react any differently.

In recent years, jawbone cancer in dogs has been on the rise, and veterinarians are at a loss to find an explanation. Perhaps a study would point to chlorinated water as the cause. Research has already found that chlorine interacts with radioactive substances in the water. In *Water Fit to Drink: A Guide to the Hidden Hazards of Drinking Water and What You Can Do to Ensure a Safe, Good-Tasting Supply for the Home*, Carol Keough explains how chlorination extensively increases the amount of plutonium that the body absorbs. Plutonium is poisonous to the body, disabling the proper production of white blood cells.

Fluoride

Fluoride is added to toothpaste and water as a preventative against dental decay. Americans consume more fluoride than those in any other country in the world. It was originally introduced because, as a byproduct of the manufacturing of aluminum, it was discovered that it could be marketed as a reinforcement for dental enamel. However, fluoride is a known poison. It has been used as a pesticide and, in concentrated form, as a rat poison that also causes the death of scores of innocent animals. Just one-tenth of an ounce of fluoride can cause death in humans. This substance was banned in many European countries and in Australia some time ago.

At 1 part per million (ppm), fluoride helps prevent tooth decay, but at 2 ppm, dental fluorosis (staining of the teeth) can occur. Research has shown that greater amounts of fluoride can cause crippling bone disorders in humans. According to the *Physicians' Desk Reference*, fluoride can have many adverse effects on humans, causing such disorders as eczema, Down syndrome, gastric distress, headaches, and mottling of the teeth. It also has been reported to exacerbate kidney disease, hypoglycemia, hormonal imbalance, birth defects, and even cancer. In 1975, Dr. Dean Burk, former head chemist of the National Cancer Institute, reported to Congress that fluoride was linked to over 10,000 cancer deaths in the United States each year. It is thought to change the genetic structure of cells and chromosomes. If humans can develop these illnesses from fluoride, think of what it can do to our comparatively smaller pets!

People brush their teeth with fluoride toothpaste, drink water with fluoride added, and are treated with fluoride at the dentist. Pets normally get fluoride only in water, unless you brush their teeth, but danger exists when fluoride amounts exceed 1 ppm. (Fluoride toothpaste can sometimes have up to 1,000 ppm.) Since pets are smaller and ingest more fluoride concentrations per body weight than humans do, the threat increases. If you have fluoride added to your water (usually city water) and your pet develops bone problems, consult with your veterinarian about fluoride poisoning.

The EPA has set a limit of 4 ppm of fluoride in drinking water. "Fluoride Health Scan," from the *Sarasota Eco Report* (Volume 4, #2, February, 1994; reprinted with permission from Acres, USA), reports that the National Academy of Sciences evaluated this situation and determined that the present limit should be an "interim" standard until more research is done. After an animal study reported a high rate of bone tumors in male rats exposed to doses of 100 ppm of fluoride, the EPA conducted a review of these standards. However, according to the *National Institute of Environmental Health Report* (1993), the EPA panel came to the conclusion that dental fluorosis (staining of the teeth) is the only condition likely to arise from consuming excess fluoride in drinking water. The handling of this situation is not comforting. What is happening to our small pets while panels are waiting for research results before they "up" the restrictions?

Lead

Most cases of canine lead poisoning are blamed on the dogs' chewing of lead-painted wood. However, there have been situations in which animals have exhibited symptoms of lead poisoning but no lead paint has been found. Veterinarians may not be identifying the culprit properly. You must test your water supply to find out whether your tap water could be a source of illness for your animal. If lead-positive results come back and you notice your pet exhibiting odd symptoms, bring this to the attention of your veterinarian so that he or she can perform a lead test on your animal.

Symptoms of lead poisoning include gastric upset, neurological dysfunction, anorexia, restlessness, and kidney disorders. Dogs also exhibit distemper-like symptoms—foaming at the mouth, growling, and chomping of jaws. The Environmental Protection Agency reports that 22 percent of large water systems in the United States exceed the lead action level—the amount at which remediation procedures are required to start—which registers at 0.015. Most of these systems are in the Northwest, Midwest, and Northeast. If you live in these areas, be sure to evaluate the presence of lead in your water with a lead-in-water test kit.

In the past, indoor plumbing consisted of lead pipes. When lead began to appear in drinking water, these pipes were replaced with copper ones. Unfortunately, it wasn't until recently that lead solder for pipes was also banned, so many copper plumbing systems still leach lead into the water. If you are on a city water system that relies on lead piping anywhere along the supply route, you are at risk even if you make sure that your own plumbing is lead-free.

Faucets, especially those that have bronze or brass fittings, may contain lead because the metals usually are mixed with a certain amount of lead substance and because it's also possible that lead solder was used during manufacturing. While the law forbids a leaching of more than half of a microgram of lead into every liter of water, *Water Technology* has reported that of twenty faucet brands tested by the University of North Carolina, nineteen leached more lead than the law allows. Manufacturers of faucets claim that they give the consumer plenty of warning, and that their faucets meet all state and federal regulations.

Regardless, you should run the water for several minutes before taking the first drink of the day, just to flush out lead.

Public water system pipes can produce unhealthy levels of lead in the water. Old service pipes and newer pipes with lead solder contribute to the contamination. The EPA states that as many as 30 million people served by 819 large and medium-sized public water systems could be drinking water with dangerously high lead levels. Water system companies are required to test for lead in houses served by lead service lines, and to notify these customers of the hazard. However, many do not adequately monitor the systems, nor do they inform their users of the hazards of lead-contaminated water. (For more information on lead poisoning, see Chapter 4.)

Bottled Water

To avoid the pollutants that contaminate tap water, many people turn to bottled water. However, the University of Tennessee Agricultural Extension Service discovered that bottled water is not necessarily safer. Bottled water is checked by the Food and Drug Administration (FDA), not the Environmental Protection Agency. The FDA tests such water only when a consumer complains, and has found that many of the manufacturers do not comply with United States drinking water standards. The organization has set standards for bottled water that regulate levels of inorganic and synthetic organic chemicals, synthetic volatile organic chemicals, some pesticides, and some PCBs (polyvinyl chlorides that are liquid wastes of plastics manufacturing and are often dispersed in water). There are no limits for other toxic pesticides or for asbestos.

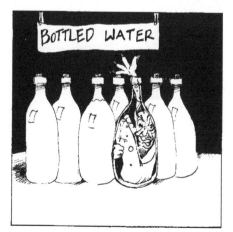

Mineral-Deficient Water

Reverse osmosis and distillation methods of water purification will remove nearly 100 percent of the dissolved solids from water. This includes the pollutants in the water, but, unfortunately, it also includes the minerals that are necessary for your pet's health. Water that has been treated by these methods has been called "dead," because it lacks the natural life-force elements.

Minerals and electrolytes are the "sparks" of life. Without the proper amounts of minerals, our bodies' defense systems cannot function properly. Electrolytes—ions such as sodium, potassium, and chloride that are needed by cells to control the electric charge and flow of water molecules across the cell membrane—are the basis of every physical and neurological function. They are used in the function and repair of all tissue, and in the utilization of amino acids. Electrolytes maintain osmotic equilibrium—the internal water balance that enables muscles and nerves to contract and expand, and wounds to heal. Neither muscles nor nerves function properly unless they are bathed in tissue fluids that contain mineral salts. The proper growth and development of the bones and organs are also dependent on electrolyte balance. Electrolytes act to increase the absorption and effects of vitamins, macrominerals, and proteins (amino acids) from food and natural supplements such as kelp, garlic, yeast, cod liver oil, and wheat germ oil. Purified water that is not supplemented with minerals and electrolytes will deprive your pet of much needed nutrition.

Well Water

Well water usually doesn't contain chlorine or fluoride, but there are no guarantees that other contaminants are not seeping into the water source. Nitrates from agricultural runoff and septic tank leakage are a good example. It is important to realize that, inside the body, nitrates can be transformed into compounds called *nitrosamines*. Studies have reported that nitrosamines cause cancer in rats.

In farm country, herbicides are used for weed control on a predetermined schedule, regardless of need. The amount of herbicides applied per acre is growing every year. When nitrates and chemicals from herbicides leach into well water, the mixing of their properties may result in even higher toxicity. Many substances are inert until they are mixed with others. Dangerous reactions and the production of completely new poisonous substances can occur.

The Solution

The first step in preventing water contamination from being a problem in your home is to avoid the use of products that can contaminate the water supply. As we have seen throughout this book, many substances, including the pesticides you may spray on your lawn and the products you may use to clean your house, can leach into the water supply and cause health problems. However, some sources of water pollution—chlorine, fluoride, lead from public supply pipes, etc.—are beyond your control. In these cases, the best way to keep your pet safe from water contamination is to give him or her water that has been filtered.

City Water

Most pollutants in city water can be removed through the use of carbon filters, reverse osmosis systems, or distillers. These filtration units are effective in removing many contaminants and are the only removal methods for toxic gases such as chloroform. The following information on these systems is gathered from *Your Health and Your House* by Nina Anderson and Albert Benoist.

Carbon filtration involves a water in/water out technique that yields the same amount of water that is received. In other words, there is no reduction of water in the purification process. The water runs through a cartridge that traps dissolved solids. The filters should be replaced every six to twelve months, according to frequency of usage and the level of contamination in the water. There are several types of carbon filtration, including *activated carbon filters,* which absorb chlorine, chloroform, pesticides, PCBs, herbicides, radon, trihalomethanes, and certain organic chemicals; *Ecolyte* (by Sterling Springs), which removes lead, in addition to the above-named contaminants; and *Amtek carbon/resin cartridges,* which eliminate the threat of all of the above, plus mercury and cadmium. Portable carbon filters are available, so that you can purify the water at hotels and other locations during your travels. You can also purchase activated carbon shower filters; chlorine mist during a shower is equally if not more toxic than drinking chlorinated water.

Reverse osmosis systems yield approximately one gallon of filtered water for every three gallons of water that enters the unit. Depending on the size of the system, these units can produce anywhere from five to one hundred gallons of purified water per day. Both carbon filters and membrane filters are used; carbon filters should be replaced every six months, while membrane filters should be changed approximately once a year. Of course, the level of water contamination and the frequency of usage will ultimately determine the proper scheduling of filter replacement. Reverse osmosis systems are capable of removing up to 98 percent of dissolved solids from the water, including arsenic; copper; fluoride; fungicides; herbicides; lead; nitrates; certain pesticides; radium; radon; sodium, and volatile organic compounds (VOCs).

Another method of water filtration is the *distillation process.* If the distiller is equipped with a carbon filter, the unit will eliminate most dissolved solids, including dirt and rust; fluoride; heavy metals; nitrates; and sodium. It will also eliminate bacteria and microorganisms. The distillation process is electrical and filters slowly; it can take up to five hours to get one gallon of distilled water.

For more information on methods of water treatment, contact the Water Quality Association. (See the Information Resources list, page 115.)

Chlorine

The best way to determine if your water source contains chlorine is to use a do-it-yourself test kit that will indicate the presence of chlorine, as well as nitrates, nitrites, iron, acidity, and hardness. If chlorine is present in your water, take precautions to keep your pet from becoming ill by giving him or her filtered water.

Water filters containing activated carbon have been proven to be effective at removing chlorine, gases such as chloroform, and hydrocarbon organic-based chemicals, including pesticides, PCBs, and trihalomethanes (chlorine byproducts). Activated carbon filters can be placed on water supply pipes at the point of use (attached to an individual faucet). These filters must be replaced periodically, as the absorptive capacity of the carbon is eventually depleted. Many filters last at least six months, depending on the level of contamination, and they are not expensive to replace.

Ozone has been used for water treatment since the eighteenth century. It is one of the best germicides available, and has the ability to destroy pathogenic organisms such as cysts, viruses, amoebas, and spores, all of which are resistant to chlorine. Unlike chlorine, ozone does not produce toxic byproducts, is not corrosive, and does not irritate the eyes. It is used primarily for industrial, commercial, and community water purification. Many cities in Europe have been using this method to treat their water for years, and the city of Los Angeles used ozone in its Olympic swimming pool. Many more American cities are now turning to ozone purification to eliminate the hazards associated with chlorination. Unfortunately, due to the political power of the chlorine industry, ozone is rarely used for home water systems.

Fluoride

If you don't want to wait until the government determines if fluoride is absolutely safe at the present limits, you can treat your drinking water by installing a reverse osmosis filtration system or a distillation system. Your pet does not need the fluoride supplied in tap water. In fact, it is safest to remove this substance from your water supply.

Lead

The only solution for the removal of lead is to use either point-of-use or whole-house filtration. The proper systems for removing lead from water are reverse osmosis, distillation, and certain types of carbon filtration. Using only granulated activated carbon (GAC) filters will not remove lead from the water. Many inexpensive, commercial point-of-use filters rely solely on GACs. If you are purchasing a filtering system, make sure that lead removal is guaranteed.

Bottled Water

Bottled water is often used as a substitute for tap water, but as you learned earlier, it is not always safer. You should not assume that bottled water is free from contamination; contact the manufacturer and request a water-test-result report. Because many contaminants can be found in their supply, most bottled water manufacturers are now running their water through reverse osmosis units before bottling. In general, bottled water is filtered, but *not* necessarily treated for parasites. Please be aware that bottled water that is untreated and has been stored for a period of time in a warm warehouse could breed bacteria.

Spring water comes from out of the ground. Unless it is routinely tested or run through a purifier, it can contain contaminants. If you are purchasing bottled spring water, research the source and inquire about the manufacturer's standards.

Mineral-Deficient Water

If you give your pet water that is treated by reverse osmosis or distillation, it is absolutely necessary to supplement his or her diet with minerals and electrolytes, either by adding them to the purified water or to your animal's food. Liquid crystalloid solutions, which contain the proper combination of trace minerals needed by the body, are the best supplements. Individual mineral supplements might not optimally treat your pet's deficiency, and incorrect dosages can upset his or her entire mineral balance. For more information, see the "Minerals," section of Chapter 8, page 98.

Well Water

If you are concerned about nitrates and/or nitrites in well water, you can purchase an over-the-counter home-test kit. For a detailed survey of all the pollutants in your water, hire a professional to perform a complete test. To the disadvantage of test accuracy, pollutants in water may come and go and it is not practical to have a survey performed frequently. Safe water is most assured by using either whole-house or point-of-use filtration. Before you purchase a filter, review your water test results with a water treatment expert so that you will know specifically what you need from a filtration unit.

Sulfur, normally found in shallow wells, is not necessarily harmful. However, its foul odor can deter pets from drinking the water, thereby leading to dehydration. If sulfur is present, carefully observe your animal to make sure that he or she is drinking enough.

Your pet relies on you to provide clean water. After all, water is the essence of life. Avoid giving your animal tap water and do not allow him or her to drink from the toilet. Tainted water will compromise your pet's immune system. Although many animals naturally lap up puddle water and will drink from just about any water source, they are not naturally immune to all of the toxins that may infest the supply. Many pollutants are a result of the unnatural methods and systems of present-day civilization. Please don't let your pet pay the price for the environmental carelessness that has contaminated much of our water.

While humans and pets are being put at risk due to contaminated subsurface water, wild animals drinking from open streams and lakes are at the mercy of toxic surface water. Pollution, acid rain, agricultural runoff, and industrial spills leach into the water. You can take part in providing a cleaner world for these creatures by helping to police the waterways, by supporting environmental organizations, and by living as nontoxically as possible.

8.
Your Pet's Health

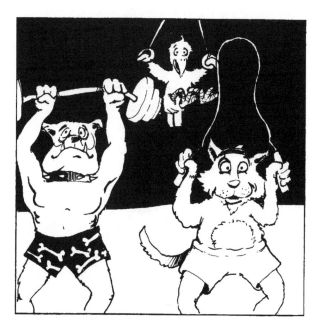

The previous chapters have offered information and
solutions concerning various threats to your pet's
health. Now we turn to proper health maintenance.
People often assume that animals' instincts lead them on the
path to adequate diet and activity. But especially considering the ways in which modern lifestyles affect natural
habits, you should not depend on your pet's inherited

lessons from the wild. The best defense against most toxins is to keep your pet's immune system at its peak; appropriate diet, supplementation, exercise, the treatment of ailments, and healthy indoor air are essential to your animal companion's well-being. This chapter discusses these topics and serves as a steppingstone for further research and awareness. Your journey toward providing a better living environment and optimal care for your pet is off to a strong start.

Diet

Many animal care professionals and pet owners now believe that commercial pet foods are about as good for pets as fast foods are for humans. The majority of these products are highly processed and, as a result, depleted of vitamins and minerals. They also contain questionable chemical additives and low-quality ingredients that have been rejected for human consump-

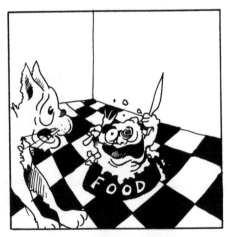

tion. Advertising claims of "complete and balanced" pet foods are based on minimum nutritional requirements designed merely for adequate health, not for *optimum* health. With foods like these, it is no wonder that so many pets become prematurely sick. However, there are a few brands that stand out as nutritionally responsible: *PetGuard*; *PHD*; and *Solid Gold*. Please refer to the Product Directory, page 117, for more information on these and other products named throughout this chapter.

Countless cat and dog owners give their animals "people food." Be discriminating in what kind of table scraps you offer your pet, for your kindness could be harming the animal. For example, if liver makes up more than 10 percent of a cat's diet, the cat may be ingesting too much vitamin A.

The result is distorted bones, gingivitis, teeth problems, and stiff joints. Also, if you feed your pet only one type of food—all beef or all chicken, for example—you may need to add supplements to his or her diet.

Some vegetarians enforce their beliefs on their pets, albeit with the best of intentions. Unfortunately, most animals do not thrive on vegetarian diets. Cats, in particular, need taurine—an amino acid-like substance found in meat and fish. Without sufficient taurine, the cat is likely to develop degeneration of the heart muscle and may also go blind. Dogs tolerate all-vegetable diets better than cats do, as dogs are able to synthesize sufficient quantities of taurine. Still, nutritionally balanced diets that include meat are best. Be sure to avoid meats and fish that have been contaminated with pesticides, hormones, and heavy metals.

Green foods are an important part of your pet's diet because of the beneficial enzymes that they add. For example, chlorophyll—a pigment found in green plants—is an internal antiseptic, cell stimulator, red blood cell builder, and rejuvenator. It relieves respiratory troubles and discomforts in the sinuses and lungs, and helps improve blood and heart conditions. The best sources of chlorophyll are alfalfa, barley grass, wheat grass, blue-green algae, and spirulina. Barley grass also contains tocopherol acid succinate, a compound that has the potential to prevent the body's immune system from breaking down as it fights off defense-crippling diseases.

Other substances that are good for your cat or dog are parsley, nutritional yeast, and cod liver oil (which contains vitamins A and D) for the immune system; garlic for digestion; nettles for the skin; burdock as a digestive cleanser; hawthorn for the heart; buchu for the bladder; oats for the nervous system; and celery seed for the muscles and joints. Products containing any of these nutrients will ultimately enhance your animal companion's health. Consult a holistic veterinarian for proper advice on your pet's diet, as these substances should be administered according to the animal's specific condition, breed, weight, age, etc. (See "Natural Healing Remedies," found later in this chapter, for more information on the health benefits of certain herbs.)

Birds, too, are at great risk of malnutrition when fed on today's commercial seed. It is important to realize that many companies use false advertising to promote their products. For example, certain feed companies claim that they offer a "complete" parrot food, yet some veterinarians argue that the minimum nutritional requirements for parrots are not known. Therefore, these companies are making unsound statements. The real proof is how healthy your bird looks and acts. Sickly birds exhibit missing feathers, poor pigmentation, extremes in weight (thinness or obesity), and weak bones. Furthermore, high-fat diets often cause wet and malodorous droppings. Birds who possess these symptoms usually have been fed seed with minimal levels of the essential fatty acids and amino acids that are necessary for the maintenance of energy. Their illnesses could be due to fillers and additives in the seed, or simply to poorly grown or rancid seeds. Another problem, especially threatening to the underdeveloped immune systems of baby birds, is microbial contamination of seed. This is usually remedied through avoiding bird food that contains animal byproducts, fish, or eggs, all of which may be tainted with harmful organisms. It is wise to ask your seed suppliers if they test for bacteria counts. For more information on proper nutrition for pet birds, contact the Hagen Avicultural Research Institute, listed in the Information Resources list, page 115. Also, read Alicia McWatters' *A Guide to a Naturally Healthy Bird*.

Many people feed the wild birds throughout the winter months, but do not think it is necessary to continue as the weather starts to warm. However, spring is a particularly critical time for birds, as their normal stores of winter seed are gone and plants are not yet producing. Please continue to feed your wild birds in the spring, as well as throughout the summer. This will make their lives easier while they are struggling to find enough food for their young. When selecting a commercial wild bird feed, look for a product that comes from organically grown plants; if seeds are collected from non-organic plants, their nutrition value is compromised. For both wild birds and caged birds, we recommend *Wings* bird food. It is the first all-natural, fortified bird food.

Supplements

Wise pet owners supplement their animals' diets. Minerals, enzymes, and essential fatty acids strengthen and support the immune system and should be a regular part of your pet's nutrition regimen. Vitamins and herbs can also prove extremely helpful in improving and maintaining your pet's health.

The administering of *vitamin* supplements is not suggested as a daily part of a healthy animal's diet. If, according to a veterinarian's advice, your pet requires vitamins, supplementation must be carefully structured around the animal's breed, age, weight, health condition, etc. Therefore, it is crucial that you consult a holistic veterinarian on this subject, as opposed to making decisions on your own. We suggest that, if vitamins are necessary, you purchase powdered supplements, which are easily mixed into the pet's food. Pill forms are likely to make your animal dread dinnertime and will upset his or her eating schedule.

Enzymes

Enzymes are catalysts for biological functions; they are the driving force behind all life processes and are responsible for keeping an animal's internal systems working. Every animal, including the human being, is born with an integral supply of enzymes. In addition, the pancreas manufactures enzymes for a multitude of purposes, one of which is food digestion. Ideally, the animal then ingests additional enzymes through diet, allowing a healthy reserve to stay intact.

As early as 1920, Dr. Edward Howell discovered the association between enzyme intake and health. He theorized that enzymes in foods are used during the process of digestion. Research indicates that most animals' digestive systems allow the food enzymes time to act before the body's own digestive process begins. This *predigestion* is important to the body's absorption of nutrients. If it is not present, then food may pass through the system without releasing its vitamins and proteins. The body's various stores of enzymes must then be diverted, leaving a diminished supply to fight disease and to perform essential bodily functions. Unfortunately, as generations go by and fewer enzymes are taken into the body because of improper diet, the stores are used up and the number of inherited enzymes decreases. This promotes degenerative disease.

Only raw or uncooked foods contain enzymes, and since almost all pet food is cooked or processed with heat, the majority of pets do not receive adequate amounts of enzymes. Literature from the Price Pottenger Foundation reports on a study of Dr. Francis Pottenger's cats. The animals were fed only cooked or processed foods. The study followed the family line of the cats and found that, over many generations, degenerative disease appeared at increasingly younger ages. Dr. Pottenger's cats acquired kidney, heart, thyroid, and gum diseases, as well as allergies, infections, and numerous other maladies. They had fewer enzymes to pass onto their offspring, leading to minimal reserves. We have seen this evidenced in the early onset of arthritic conditions in cats. Enzymes enhance the absorption of nutrients and assure that these nutrients enter the cells. Without absorption, the body becomes imbalanced and cannot eliminate toxins. These toxins may lodge in the joints and result in pain and swelling. Your pet might live as long as previous generations in the family line, but quality of life suffers.

When the immune system is under stress, it uses enzymes to maintain body functions. Enzymes are lost through sickness, pregnancy, anxiety, extreme weather conditions, urine, and feces. Unless these stores are replaced, your pet's immune system will be compromised. (This is also true for humans, evident through the fact that our younger generations are developing earlier cases of heart disease, arthritis, and susceptibility to allergies.) You should supplement your pet's diet with nutritional enzymes if he or she depends on canned or dried food. For cats and dogs, we recommend Prozyme Product's *Prozyme*. Birds who are fed raw food or seed diets do not need enzyme supplementation. However, if you nourish your bird on cooked-food mash, then supplements are likely to be necessary. In all cases, please consult a holistic veterinarian for advice that is specific to your animal.

Essential Fatty Acids

Essential fatty acids (EFAs) provide health benefits that aid in the *prevention* of disease and illness and, therefore, are an integral part of health maintenance. Dr. Michael Gazsi, N.D., is a strong believer in EFA supplementation. The following passage is from one of his lectures at the Natural Health Center in East Canaan, Connecticut:

> Another often overlooked nutrient that is essential to life is the EFA (essential fatty acid). These fats, known as omega-3 and omega-6, cannot be made by the body and have to be ingested through food. Commercial pet foods are very poor sources of EFAs. Oils containing EFAs are easily damaged by heat, light, and oxygen. The heat used to make sure the food contains no bacteria, and the long exposure of the oils to air and light in storage, cause the remaining EFAs to be damaged to the point where they are no longer beneficial. In fact, they become *trans fats*, which are detrimental to the animals' health by inhibiting the normal oils' function in the body. It has long been known that essential fatty acid deficiency causes dry flaky skin, increased susceptibility to cutaneous infections, and hair loss in dogs. Linoleic acid [the primary omega-6 fatty acid] supplementation can lessen the severity of the condition and can correct the fatty acid imbalance in the skin.
>
> Omega-3 and omega-6, properly balanced in their unadulterated forms, are necessary for the building blocks of membranes in every cell in the body; for energy metabolism, as they are used to make a hormone family called *prostaglandins*; for cardiovascular health; for bowel and immune function; and as a preventative for cancers, diabetes, arthritis, asthma, all inflammatory tissue conditions, skin conditions, impaired visual function, and fertility problems, to name a few. With these in mind, it would be wise to supplement the animal's diet with EFAs on a daily basis.

EFAs can be ingested through oils. Cold-pressed flaxseed oil, fish oils (including cod liver oil), borage oil, evening primrose oil, sunflower oil, and safflower oil are excellent if the product truly has been cold-pressed in dark containers. Unfortunately, most of today's cold-pressed products are heated at some point to control shelf life.

Flaxseed, if eaten as a whole grain or ground into a powder, is an excellent alternative to oils. It also is a healthy source of protein, since it contains eight amino acids, complex carbohydrates to regulate protein and fat metabolism, vitamins, minerals, and roughage to remove toxins and bile cholesterol via elimination.

For EFA supplementation in cat and dog diets, we recommend *Animal Essentials*, by Merritt Naturals. If your pet has difficulty with pills, try *Fortified Flax*, which consists of powdered (ground) flaxseed that can be added to pet food. Also, NUPRO contains EFAs, among other ingredients, in a powdered product that becomes a gravy-like mixture when combined with water. Birds get essential fatty acids in seeds and nuts, but you can further enhance your pet bird's nutrition by supplementing with flax oil, flax meal, or evening primrose. We suggest *Fortified Flax* for birds, as well.

Minerals

Today's animals and humans have a marked disadvantage over creatures from the past—we are lacking proper amounts of trace minerals. During the Ice Age, mineral-rich soil was deposited over the planet, but erosion and chemical farming methods have caused depletion of trace minerals in topsoil, as well as in the plants that are grown from the soil. Furthermore, while water used to be a healthy source of trace minerals, the filtering processes that cleanse water also eliminate what minerals are left. When we lack adequate amounts of trace minerals, our bodies' defense systems cannot function correctly. As a result, toxins accumulate and we become increasingly susceptible to infection. Likewise, mineral-deficient pets who are exposed to toxins are much more likely to develop disease than pets with the proper amounts of nutrients. Animals lacking sufficient supplies of copper, iron, selenium, and other minerals have been found to have an increased risk of cancer. In addition, the drugs and vitamins given to mineral-deficient, sick animals are often useless. Vitamins are fortifiers; they control the body's use of minerals. In the absence of minerals, the vitamins have no function. Putting minerals back into your pet's diet is essential.

Crystalloid minerals are minerals that bypass the digestive process and are absorbed directly into cell walls, strengthening the immune system. In September of 1991, Brian Thompson, a retired horse trainer, administered crystalloid minerals to race horses in upstate New York. He used a liquid version, as the horses had rejected a dry electrolyte formula. A marked improvement was seen in the animals' behavior. The horses were much more alert, less nervous, and less jumpy. Their coats improved; one horse with an injury-induced patch of skin that had been bare for two years actually began to grow back the hair. Muscle soreness and stiffness disappeared, and the horses' racing abilities improved. This example illustrates the significance of trace minerals when it comes to an animal's physical and mental health.

If your pet's diet lacks trace minerals, he or she is not likely to be converting proteins properly. This is important since most pet foods are meat-based. You may be feeding your animal a good amount of food, but he or she might be nutritionally starving if the body is unable to process the food. Properly balanced *minerals with electrolytes* are a wise investment, as they will help keep your pet's immune system working correctly. Purchase liquid crystalloid minerals, which contain the necessary combination. Supplementing your pet's diet with individual minerals may not be the best way of attacking a health problem; if dosages are not correct, you might be harming the animal's mineral balance, instead of improving it.

The simplest way to add minerals to your pet's diet is to dribble liquid supplements into the water dish. (The dosage of liquid crystalloid minerals is one drop per pound of the animal's weight.) It is important to avoid colloidal minerals. They are too large to get absorbed by the cell and end up floating around in the vascular system, where they could deposit themselves in joints and in the urinary tract, causing serious health problems. *PetLyte*, manufactured by Naturopathic Research, contains a full complement of trace minerals that will sufficiently supplement an animal's diet.

Supporting a pet's immune system with supplements will result in fewer visits to the veterinarian and will allow the animal a longer, healthier life span. But keep in mind that even supplements can be manufactured with low-quality ingredients and potentially allergenic substances, such as brewer's yeast, milk, wheat, artificial flavors, and dyes, all of which can cause scratching, skin problems, and diarrhea. Therefore, be sure to read labels carefully and choose products wisely. In addition to supplement forms of enzymes, essential fatty acids, and minerals, consider adding the following natural substances to your pet's diet: nutritional yeast; Norwegian kelp; spirulina; sprouted barley; wheat grass; yucca; bee pollen; essential fatty acids in the form of flax, borage, and lecithin; garlic; acidophilus; rice bran; alfalfa; freeze dried bone; carrots; fish meal; and nettles. Your pet's immune system and healing capacities will benefit greatly. Information on herbal remedies for specific conditions is provided later in this chapter. And for a more detailed look at pet nutrition, read *Super Nutrition for Animals (Birds Too!)* by Nina Anderson, Howard Peiper, and Alicia McWatters.

Exercise

Exercise is as important to your pet as it is to you. "Couch potato" pets are at similar risk of heart ailments as "couch potato" humans, especially if their diets contain high amounts of fat. Indoor pets are usually overfed and rarely exercised. Animals, especially dogs, will beg for food. If their demands are constantly met, they are likely be plagued with obesity. Putting an animal on a more rigorous health plan may seem cruel when those pitiful eyes watch you eat your succulent dinner, but it is probably necessary. Before implementing any

Administering Remedies and Supplements

Sometimes the biggest challenge in providing optimal healthcare for a pet is simply figuring out how to administer a remedy or a supplement. Some pets are very resistant to pills and extremely clever when it comes to detecting substances that are "hidden" in their food. Stephen Tobin, D.M.V., of Meriden, Connecticut, offers some helpful advice on this subject.

Once you have determined what remedy or supplement to give your pet, you then have to administer it effectively. Homeopathic remedies, which come in pellets, are easy; open the dog's mouth and toss a pellet on the back of the tongue, or open the cat's mouth and drop five to ten "number 10" granules on the tongue. If this method is repeatedly unsuccessful, pellets can be crushed between two spoons and the powder sprinkled on the tongue or rubbed on the gums. Do not put homeopathic medicines in food. They need to be absorbed over the mucous membranes, and the fat in food may coat the pellets and prevent this from happening. Remedies may also be given in water—either in drinking water or dissolved and given by syringe or dropper. This is an especially effective method when treating birds.

Supplements, herbal remedies, and medications may be a little more difficult to give to your pet. Of all the housepets, dogs have the easiest time with pills. Put the pill in a small piece of something that the dog likes, such as cheese, meat, or bread. My favorite is cream cheese, as it is easy to mold, tastes good to most dogs, and doesn't stick to the roof of the mouth like peanut butter. Liquid extracts, including teas, can be squirted into the dog's mouth with a syringe or mixed with food or a treat. Some dogs will even drink teas out of a bowl. Powdered remedies can also be placed in the pet's food, combined with a treat, or stirred into water and administered with a syringe.

Cats are more of a problem. They hate alcohol, so be sure to purchase only glycerine extracts. Liquids and powders can sometimes by given in cream or half and half, in tuna water, or in chicken broth. Some solid remedies can be mixed into the foods or treats that the cat especially likes. If all else fails, powder the pill, mix it with *Nutrical*, and smear it on the top of the cat's paw. In cleaning this off, the cat will ingest the substance. You could, of course, try to open the cat's mouth, throw the pill as far back as possible, clamp the mouth shut, and stroke the throat, which sometimes works. If you are fast, you can squirt a syringeful of water into the cat's mouth after tossing in the pill, so that the cat will swallow to avoid choking. In either case, the head must by held horizontally. Like us, cats cannot swallow with their heads tilted all the way back. Be aware that this brute force method has its problems: the stress on the cat tends to depress the immune system, slowing down the healing process; and after the second pilling, the cat will hide whenever you approach and make the effective administering of a treatment even more difficult!

As recommended with homeopathic medicines, birds will often accept remedies and supplements in their food or in their water—teas can be substituted for the bird's drinking water, or glycerine extracts can be added to the water. Try to avoid alcohol extracts. For an easier time with non-liquid substances, open the capsules or crush the pills and mix the powder with food or treats such as fruit, honey, raw meat, or anything else the bird might eat readily.

Of course, some animals are more difficult to treat than others. Sometimes pets will absolutely refuse to eat or drink if they identify unpleasant substances in their food and water. Try not to upset your pet's eating habits too severely. You may have to experiment with several forms before you find one that can be administered successfully. The key is to have patience and persistence, and to talk with your veterinarian concerning any advice or alternatives that he or she may have.

dietary regime for your pet, you should contact your veterinarian for advice. And as you concentrate on proper feeding, don't forget the importance of daily exercise.

When you exercise your pet, you should be conscious of the animal's athletic ability. Dogs who are in tiptop shape may be able to jog seven miles with you, but if your specific pet is not used to exercise, permanent damage could result. Animals, like humans, have to build up gradually to rigorous exercise, so be aware of 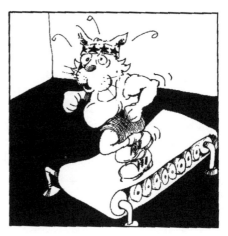 your pet's limits. Do not let your dog overdo; many dogs desire to please their owners at any cost, and will try to keep up with the bicycle or the runner. Ensure that house cats receive adequate exercise by playing with them often and supplying them with space to climb, crawl, and leap. Caged birds should be allowed to fly around the house, under close supervision, as often as possible. However, keep in mind that your bird is in danger of other pets, human visitors, cleaning products, and food stuffs that are left open. Therefore, take any necessary precautions.

Natural Healing Remedies

Selecting a remedy for a pet's illness should be left to the expertise of a veterinarian, but the following treatments are drug-free options that some doctors may not even consider. We offer them for educational purposes only. You should discuss these natural alternatives with your pet's healthcare professional.

Arthritis and Rheumatism

Arthritis is characterized by the discomfort and swelling that results from inflamed joints. Rheumatism afflicts the bones, joints, muscles, nerves, and tendons, causing stiffness, pain, and disability. These conditions affect cats and dogs in the same ways that they affect humans. (As far as we know, birds do not suffer from arthritic disorders.) Luckily, there are several natural remedies that relieve symptoms of arthritis and rheumatism. Alfalfa is high in chlorophyll and nutrients, and it helps to alkalize the body; the anti-rheumatic effect is probably due to alfalfa's high nutritive value. It is normally best to mix alfalfa with flax and other nutrients and put it in your pet's food. A warm paste of rosemary leaves or a hot compress of rosemary tea can soothe arthritic joints. Garlic reduces arthritic and rheumatic pain; use one-half to three cloves with each meal. Also, we recommend Kyo-

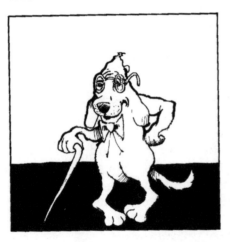

Green's *Kyolic*, an odorless, aged garlic that is available in liquid form. An oat straw bath is useful for relief of joint pain. Nettles promote anti-inflammatory actions that reduce swelling and discomfort. Yucca has been used to manage the pain of soft tissue inflammation; it is an excellent anti-inflammatory and has been proven to be a very safe and effective substitute for steroid-based medications. Parsley sprinkled into your pet's meal will strengthen your pet's immune system, especially cats, thus giving the animal an advantage in combating chronic diseases. Finally, couchgrass (also known as dog grass, twitchgrass, and quickgrass) and lavender are helpful treatments for humans suffering from rheumatism, and very well might help your pet.

Bee Stings

Fat lips and swollen noses are common for animals that find amusement in chasing bees. If your pet gets stung, aloe vera,

either fresh from a houseplant or in bottled juice form, can help to relieve the discomfort. Lavender and eucalyptus oils also reduce pain and swelling. The most effective treatment is determined by the type of sting. Sodium bi-carbonate (baking soda) dissolved in ice water is a good treatment for regu-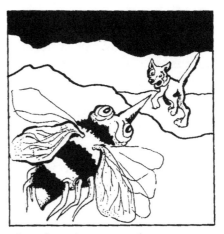
lar bee stings. If you know that the sting came from a wasp, apply thyme vinegar as an antidote.

Bites, Cuts, and Bruises

Active animals get their share of cuts and bruises. And it is not uncommon for a pet who spends a lot of time outdoors to get bitten by another animal. If not properly treated, a bite wound can become an abscess. Echinacea is an antibacterial herb that assists in the prevention of infection and stimulates the animal's immune system. Witch hazel, used topically, has an astringent action that stops bleeding and reduces inflammation and bruising. Diluted woundwort cleanses wounds and provides relief when used in a compress to cover the sore. A cloth containing a warm paste of comfrey also serves as a healing remedy, especially for deep wounds. Diluted calendula, in lotion form, is helpful for cuts and bites that have already closed; it stimulates healing and reduces pain and inflammation. Be careful *not* to apply calendula to open wounds, as it may result in premature scabbing and prevent an abscess from draining. The yucca plant, if used topically, supports tissue healing and reduces scarring. Arnica relieves bruises and sprains. We also recommend a *Five Flower Combination Formula* as a topical healing agent for your pet's injured area. Several companies make versions of this product.

Diarrhea and Digestive Problems

If you find your pet suffering from diarrhea, there are a number of natural remedies that can be of help. Capsicum is a natural stimulant for arresting diarrhea and dysentery. Garlic disinfects the digestive tract and assists in the restoration of friendly bacteria. Barberry stimulates the liver and promotes the flow of bile, which can return the bowel to normal. Try putting these natural substances in your pet's food. If he or she will not eat, then look for liquid forms and administer them orally.

There are several herbal teas that aid digestion, including teas made from caraway seed, gentian, and yucca. Also, chamomile, which is safe for all animals, is an excellent nerve relaxant, making it especially useful in treating digestive problems caused by anxiety. It reduces gas and comforts the digestive system. Peppermint oil soothes the stomach lining, subdues the urge to vomit, and also lessens gas.

Some herbs, such as dandelion and fennel, are known as stomachic herbs. They are usually bitter in flavor and are known to help promote and improve appetite and digestion. Burdock root has a soothing, alkalizing effect on the stomach and the intestines. Syrup made from the powdered bark of the slippery elm tree is highly recognized for its help with digestion. Couchgrass leaves are much sought after by many kinds of animals as a spring tonic; dogs and cats eat these leaves to promote vomiting or as a laxative. Birds and poultry eat the seeds for treatment of bladder ailments, gallstones, and constipation. The silica content of couchgrass also helps to strengthen teeth, beaks, and claws.

Black walnut expels internal parasites and tapeworms. For hairballs in cats, administer a combination of liquid chlorophyll with aloe vera juice or with psyllium, licorice root, and hibiscus flowers. If your pet has simple constipation and gas, try giving him or her a little *Carboveg* (vegetable charcoal). Finally, many animal specialists recognize the yucca plant for its stool deodorizer properties; mixing yucca into your pet's food can reduce the odors of his or her excretions.

Pets and "People Medicine"

It is extremely frustrating to see a pet in discomfort, and sometimes it is tempting to reach into the medicine cabinet and pull out a pill that works for us. However, these good intentions can cause bad reactions. Irreversible damage or death can result from giving pets medications that are manufactured for humans. Do not give drugs to your animal unless you are following the directions of your pet's doctor. Herbal and homeopathic remedies are not as risky, but still should be prescribed by a holistic veterinarian.

Human over-the-counter pain relievers occasionally are used in veterinary medicine, but, again, they should be given only according to the specific advice and directions of a veterinarian. Tylenol is generally safe for people, but small animals (cats and small dogs) do not have the ability to detoxify the drug after ingestion. It can cause destruction of red blood cells and tissue cells. Signs of poisoning include salivation, vomiting, weakness, and abdominal pain. As little as one tablet (325 milligrams) can trigger these symptoms, and two tablets can kill a small animal. Generally, larger animals are affected by larger doses.

Sometimes veterinarians prescribe aspirin, ibuprofen, phenylbutazone, and other NSAIDs (nonsteroid anti-inflammatory drugs) for pain relief. If administered in doses that are too large or for extended periods of time, the animal can develop stomach ulcers. In addition, these drugs indirectly decrease the blood flow to vital organs, particularly the kidneys, resulting in dysfunction. Two regular strength aspirin in a small dog can cause clinical signs of poisoning. Cats are even more sensitive and should not be given aspirin at all.

Muscle Spasms and Pain

Muscle discomfort can occur for a variety of reasons. Unfortunately, your pet cannot articulate how severe the problem is, or if there are additional problems, so it is best to contact a veterinarian when your pet appears debilitated. If you are confident that your animal is suffering from a muscle pull, strain, spasm, or the like, there are several natural treatments that can soothe the pain. Cayenne, fennel, lavender, and sage are known to relieve muscle spasms. Apply these herbs topically. Oats serve as a tonic, particularly for animals that exhibit twitching, tremors, or paralysis. If your pet will not eat plain oats, try mixing them into his or her food. For muscle pain, add one teaspoon of rosemary to a cup of boiling water and cool. Then add one to two drops of hazelnut or lavender oil, and work the mixture into the affected area.

Respiratory Problems

A loving pet owner hates the thought of his or her animal companion suffering from congested lungs or breathing discomfort. Fortunately, there are ways to trigger relief. Anise helps to remove excess mucus. Comfrey supplements also can be administered as an expectorant to remove mucus from the respiratory tract. Garlic has antiviral properties and is known for its effectiveness in treating lung ailments. Once ingested, the oils in garlic are excreted through the respiratory tract and are good for reducing bronchitis. Coltsfoot is an antispasmodic and expectorant with anti-inflammatory properties, due to its zinc content; it is useful in treating cases of bronchitis and cough. White horehound combines well with coltsfoot, as it dilates the airways and helps to loosen mucus. Treatments that include schizandra relieve coughing, wheezing, and asthma. Some of these above-mentioned respiratory remedies are best administered as warm liquids. Others can be purchased in supplement form. Consult a holistic veterinarian or an animal herbologist for more information.

Skin Disorders

Dry, itchy skin is an indication of many problems, and animals suffering from this problem often have bladder inflammation and pain, as well. Skin conditions are likely to be manifestations of internal illnesses. To offer your pet relief, make an infusion of sarsaparilla rootstock in one cup of near-boiling water, strain, and orally administer this remedy proportionally—from two teaspoons for a small animal, to up to six tablespoons for a large dog—three times daily. Burdock root is cooked like a carrot and used as a blood purifier; this treatment may help to correct underlying problems. Yucca, given orally as an herbal supplement, is effective in reducing the itch response in allergic animals. Topical application of calendula also proves helpful.

Stress and Emotional Disorders

Flower remedies are especially useful in treating stress and emotional disorders in all types and sizes of animals. In liquids or in creams, they can be used as an immediate solution for any situation that is stressing or traumatizing the animal, including car sickness. Try using impatiens for uptight, impatient, irritable animals; mimulus for timid animals afraid of known things such as water, thunder, and riding in cars; aspen for animals who are fearful of the unknown, suspicious and panicked at their surroundings and circumstances; chestnut bud for animals who have difficulty learning lessons during training, to help correct bad habits and negative repetitive behavior; olive for exhaustion resulting from trauma or prolonged sickness; and Star of Bethlehem for trauma or grief, or for animals who have been injured or abused.

Flower remedies also work well for reducing the pain and swelling of skin disorders, insect bites, burns, bruises, and sprains.

Urinary Tract Disorders

Animals frequently lick their private parts and strain to urinate. These are often symptoms of a urinary tract infection that is constricting the urethra and causing a pinching or burning sensation. The infection can be caused by too much ash in dried pet foods or by a bacteria. Several herbs are successful in treating this condition. Barberry has astringent and antiseptic qualities that soothe and strengthen the urinary tract. Buchu helps to dissolve urinary crystals and wash gravel through the urinary tract by increasing the flow of fluids and, thus, promoting urination. Parsley tea provides the same benefits as buchu, and can soothe the irritated area in the urinary tract. Mugwort and gravel oak are also agents of relief from urinary tract disorders.

Healthy Indoor Air

Healthy air is fundamental to your pet's well-being. This book has discussed the dangers resulting from a lack of ventilation and a poorly monitored indoor environment. Toxins remain airborne as long as your house is shut tight, and risks increase during the heating and air conditioning seasons. Air treatment and air exchange are very important to the prevention and treatment of illness. Simply suspecting that your pet is being poisoned by indoor air, or giving him or her oral antidotes under the advice of the National Poison Control Center or a veterinarian, will not keep problems from recurring. You must take care of the problem at the source.

Safer Air

Animals that are confined to indoor environments are susceptible to airborne aggravants. They can develop allergies and respiratory conditions, sometimes at higher rates than humans because they are closer to the floor, where much of the dust accumulates. Forced air systems blow dust and toxins around. Bacteria often breed in the ducts and may cause further illness. If you have one of these systems in your home, have the ducts cleaned each year before the heating or air conditioning season begins. Hot water and electric baseboard heaters are much cleaner, but they still toss toxins around as the air moves and the heat rises. These systems can even fry the dust that lands on the hot pipes, releasing additional toxins into the air. We suggest a safer alternative: overhead electric radiant panels.

Overhead electric radiant panels produce allergy-free heat and promote healthy air. The solid-state panels warm *objects*, not the air. This heating method keeps the heat down low where you need it, similar to the effect that you would get if you stood in the sun. Animals don't mind sleeping on the floor, as it is usually kept warm. Since the panels are face-mounted to the ceiling, there is no chance for dust to burn on them, and because air circulation is kept to a minimum, there is less airborne dust for pets to breathe.

As discussed in the first chapter of this book, air treatment is an absolute must for well-insulated houses. Unless you have furnished your home with natural products, you can be sure that toxic fumes from carpets, stuffed furniture, new drapes, or paint will be present. If these airborne hazards are not removed, you and your pets may become ill. There are many different types of air filtration devices that remove a variety of pollutants. Please refer to "Types of Air Treatment Units," page 20, for descriptions of several systems.

Ionic Information

Ions play an important role in the well-being of animals (including people). For example, before a thunderstorm, animals exhibit nervous and jittery behavior; after the storm passes, they seem to calm down. This is due to the fact that, before the storm, there is a high concentration of positive ions in the air. These positive ions come from friction, the atmosphere, dust, and pollution, and heavy accumulations tend to over-stimulate animals. Once the storm cleans the air through electrical discharge, negative ions are produced and a sense of calm prevails. If pets are exposed to prolonged periods of positive ions, they can develop behavioral changes and breathing difficulties.

Permanent press and synthetic fabrics carry the common "static cling," which results when positive ions interact with the negatively charged ground. Similarly, animals become statical when their fur is "electrified" in dry indoor atmospheres. Pets who are exposed to high static electricity levels for extended periods of time exhibit signs of depression or become irritable due to an excess of positive ions. The use of a negative ionizer can avoid these effects; the moisture created by a humidification process provides a more comfortable environment for your pet.

In recent years, thousands of experiments have been performed concerning the effects of positive and negative ions, which are believed to be absorbed through the lungs and to affect metabolic and glandular systems. The full moon causes a proliferation of positive ions in the air; animals may become anxious, restless, and more vocal. Negative ions are reported to create the opposite effect, allowing the body to function better. Europeans have observed the effects of positive ions in their "Witches' Winds." Fred Soyka's *The Ion Effect* explains that these winds, which blow down from mountains at certain periods in the seasons, usher an increase in traffic accidents, hospital patient deaths, suicides, and domestic violence. Through their use of chemical-based materials, manufacturers of building products are contributing to ion upsets in our homes that are similar to the effects of the "Witches' Winds." Furthermore, buildings with forced air systems create harmful positive ions because metal pipes, blowers, filters, and ducts strip the air of negative ions before it reaches its destination. This is especially evident in skyscrapers. The American Broadcasting Company has recognized behavioral changes in employees as a result of positive ionization, and has equipped its New York headquarters with ion control devices. Philco and Emerson Electric already have ion-control air conditioning systems on the market, with other manufacturers following.

Ions have been the subject of many medical studies that indicate that patients have improved recovery, less pain, better moods, and reduced reactions to allergens when negative ions are present. Negative ions also have a biological effect on bacteria and, in killing these germs, help clean the air. Installing a negative ionizer in conjunction with an air filtering device can reduce or eliminate the effects of positive ions and keep pets calmer and healthier. Aviaries report that air treatment devices with negative ion generators have kept birds from picking their feathers and pacing in their cages.

Every pet deserves to live in a home with clean, refreshing air. Between modern building materials, pollution, and the natural electrical properties of the environment, your pet must fight a tough battle against unhealthy conditions. You can make that daily challenge a lot easier by installing a simple air treatment device.

Our animal companions continually offer us unconditional love and support. Their endearing presence should not be rewarded with anything but matched loyalty and concern. Many of the dangers discussed in this book are threats to which we have unknowingly subjected our animals. Education on these issues demands greater responsibility, but also allows us to express our love more fully. Hopefully, this book has started you on your journey toward providing a healthier, more comfortable home for your pet.

Information Resources

The following organizations and publications will be of help in further educating yourself on pet health issues. They are very capable sources that will contribute to providing exceptional care for your animal companion.

Books, Magazines, and Newsletters

Anderson, Nina, Alicia McWatters, and Howard Peiper, Dr. *Super Nutrition for Animals (Birds Too!).* East Canaan, CT: Safe Goods Publishing, 1997.

McWatters, Alicia. *A Guide to a Naturally Healthy Bird.* East Canaan, CT: Safe Goods Publishing, 1997.

Gardens Alive *(magazine)*
5100 Schenley Place
Lawrenceburg, IN 47025
(812) 537–8650

Animal Tails Newsletter
Safe Goods
PO Box 36
East Canaan, CT 06024
(888) 217–7233

Holistic Veterinarian Directory

American Holistic Veterinary
Medical Association
2214 Old Emmorton Road
Bel Air, MD 21014
(410) 569–0795

(This service will provide you with names of veterinarians in your area who specialize in holistic approaches to diet.)

Organizations

Hagen Avicultural
Research Institute
PO Box 490
Rigaud, Quebec
Canada JOP 1PO

Water Quality Association
4151 Naperville Road
Lisle, IL 60532
(708) 505–0160

Poison Control Center

National Animal Poison Control Center
1717 South Philo Road
Urbana, IL 61802
(217) 333–2053

For emergency calls:

To have the entire call charged directly to your phone bill, dial 1–900–680–0000; the cost is $20 for the first five minutes, and $2.95 for each additional minute.
To pay a flat rate of $30 per case, billed to your credit card, dial 1–800–548–2423 or 1–888–4–ANI–HELP.

(Some veterinary pharmaceutical, flea control product, and agricultural chemical companies will pay for the cost of calls that are related to their products.)

Product Directory

In order to make your home a safe place for your pet and your entire family, it is necessary to become a careful consumer. A variety of health-oriented and environmentally responsible products are available. We recommend the below-listed items. To find out where you can purchase a specific product, contact the manufacturer; a phone number and/or address is given at the conclusion of each summary.

Air Treatment Units

Air Cleaners from Austin. These units provide whole-house or whole-kennel air cleaning through an eighty-square-foot HEPA (high efficiency particulate arrestor) filter and fifteen pounds of carbon filtration. This unit removes dust, most gases, and bacteria down to .3 microns as the internal fan draws air through the machine. Aquarius Health, 7220 Porter Road, Niagara Falls, NY 14304; (716) 298–4686.

Ozone Purifiers by Panda. The Panda is a practical, small, lightweight ozone generator with negative ions that is useful in kennels and aviaries to prevent skin disorders and allergies. It will eliminate pet odors, kill bacteria, and neutralize cat dander and harmful air contamination caused by indoor pollution. There are no filters to change. Quantum Electronics, 110 Jefferson Boulevard, Warwick, RI 02888; (800) 966-5575.

Silent Air Treatment by Clearveil. Developed in Japan to treat children with infantile asthma and people with allergies, the Clearveil electronic air cleaner operates silently, and works by releasing negative ions that attach themselves to airborne particles. It then attracts these contaminants to the unit with a positively charged collection sheet, which is easily changed each month. Excellent for odors, viruses, smoke, animal dander, mold fragments, and bacteria. Clearveil Corp., 1660 17th Street, Suite 200, Denver, CO 80202; (800) 531-6662.

Cleaning Products and Air Fresheners

A Botanical Solution to Odor Pollution. The Hygenaire is an all-natural, safe, nontoxic, odorless air freshener and deodorizer that uses vegetable and citrus extracts. It contains no cover-up scents, harmful fragrances, or petrochemicals. Within the housing is a small fan that continually evaporates the solution into the air, reducing pet area and litter box odors. The solution treats an area of 240-square-feet and lasts for six weeks or longer. Allergy Alternatives, 440 Godfrey Drive, Windsor, CA 95492; (707) 838–1514.

Natural Zeolite Minerals for Odor. The minerals in Odorzout are mined in Arizona and have a honeycomb-like structure with pores that absorb and trap unpleasant odors. Odorzout is great in litter boxes, deters flea and tick infestation, may be sprinkled on dirt pet runs and in pet houses, and is effective in removing skunk odors from your pet. It takes urine odors out of carpet, padding, and flooring, and since it contains no chemicals or perfumes, it is safe for both people and pets. No Stink, 6020 West Bell Road #E101, Glendale, AZ 85308; (800) 88–STINK.

Old-Fashioned, Unscented Safe Soaps. Coastline Products makes a variety of safe alternatives to laundry and dishwashing detergents, carpet shampoos, and fabric stain removers. They are biodegradable and contain no formaldehyde, fragrance, phosphates, dye, or harmful preservatives. They are nontoxic if swallowed in diluted form. Coastline Products, PO Box 6397, Santa Ana, CA 92706; (800) 554–4111.

Safe Cleaners and Deodorizers. Dr. Harvey's Pet Safe Products are nontoxic, biodegradable, unscented, cruelty-free, and earth-friendly. The All-Purpose Clean is safe for kennels, cages, litter boxes, pet toys, and so on. Aquarium Safe Glass Clean eliminates scum and deposits on aquarium glass and also works on home windows, mirrors, and acrylic surfaces. Carpet and Upholstery Clean requires no vacuuming, rinsing, or waiting for carpets to dry. Fresh Air and Fresh Fish are air deodorizers and water purifiers. Nature Pure Products, Inc., PO Box 14088, South Lake Tahoe, CA 96151; (800) 736–8122.

Flea and Tick Treatments

Flea and Tick Powders. Earth-safe, natural alternatives to harsh, potentially toxic chemicals and synthetic substitutes are the responsible way to protect your pet. Natural Animal, Inc. offers a pet care line that includes herbal shampoos, collars, natural pyrethrin-based flea and tick powders, vitamins, yeast and garlic supplements, and biodegradable, flushable litter. Their home care line includes diatomaceous earth and natural pyrethrin-based insect powders. Natural Animal, Inc., 7000 U.S. 1 North, St. Augustine, FL 32085; (800) 274–7387.

One-Year Flea Control. Terminator borate product (considered benign by the U.S. EPA) eliminates fleas for one year without toxic chemicals. Also available is Terminator "Ladybugs for Fleas," beneficial nematodes that eat flea larvae, thus breaking the flea cycle in your yard. Terminator also has Mega Pet Dip for pets (safe for even puppies and kittens) and Yard and Kennel pure eucalyptus powder, for those difficult areas. Terminator, PO Box 11436, Costa Mesa, CA 92627; (800) 242–9966.

Healthcare Products for Illnesses, Injuries, and Skin Disorders

Advanced Pet Healthcare. Arthritis Care for Dogs is the first natural topical pain relieving lotion for arthritis, hip dysplasia, muscle sprains, and strains. Skin Care for Dogs, a natural lotion, will heal even the worst skin condition within five days. Sun Spot, pet sunblock spray with an SPF of 15, protects from harmful UVA/UVB rays and prevents bleaching and discoloration of pets' coats. Also available is Bug Out, a natural nontoxic insect spray that repels fleas, ticks, and other biting insects. BioChemics Inc., 7 Faneuil Hall, Boston, MA 02109; (800) PETS–NOW.

Allergenic Skin Care. Commercial pet shampoos can cause skin irritation and other problems. Espree has formulated effective grooming shampoos and conditioners with no detergents, insecticides, or harmful drying or coat burning agents; they are formulated to prevent the growth of potentially dangerous bacteria, fungi, and other microorganisms. Their products can help relieve flea bite dermatitis, itching, other skin problems, and fur matting and tangling. Espree Animal Products, 6015 Commerce Drive, Suite 400, Irving, TX 75063; (800) 328–1317.

Formula for Allergies and Skin. BIO-COAT is a concentrated biotin feed supplement for dogs and cats that is enriched with other vitamins and minerals in a base of primary dried yeast (not brewer's yeast). It is good for dry skin, dull thinning coats, and scratching problems. BIO-COAT can be given to pets with allergies as a safe, effective, and inexpensive nutritional adjunct to prednisone and cortisone. It contains no artificial colors, flavors, or preservatives. Nickers International, Ltd., 12 Schubert Street, Department B, Staten Island, NY 10305; (800) 642–5377.

Home-Study on Remedies. For information on homeopathic and natural remedies, Advanced Animal Concepts for Alternative Solutions offers a myriad of videos, books, and home-study courses on the following subjects: herbs, flower remedies, gem essence, acupressure, chiropractic, massage, sports therapies, working dogs, and other alternative therapies. Advanced Animal Concepts for Alternative Solutions, 2152 Hazlitt Drive, Houston, TX 77032; (800) 228–8768.

Homeopathic Remedies. HomeoPet offers 100-percent natural homeopathic pet treatments for anxiety, arthritis, cough, flea dermatitis, gastroenteritis, hot spot dermatitis, miliary eczema (male and female), sinusitis, skin trauma and seborrhea, trauma, urinary infections, and incontinence. They all are FDA-registered, cruelty-free, and contain no chemical residue. A safe alternative to injections and drugs, these remedies are formulated by veterinarians for cats and dogs (not for human consumption). HomeoPet, Westhampton Beach, NY 11978–0147; (800) 556–0738.

Mineral and Herb Skin Spray. Skin-Aide is the first pet skin healing and nutrient spray for rebuilding of the skin. It provides relief from itchy and patchy skin, infections, fungus, and other conditions. Due to its crystalloid nature, it penetrates rapidly to the deepest skin layers with minerals and a unique ionically bound blend of five herbs. Improvement of hair growth and thicker, shinier coats can be expected. Naturopathic Research Labs, Inc., PO Box 7594, North Port, FL 34287; (800) 326–5772.

Natural Medicines Without Side Effects. Dr. Goodpet offers natural homeopathic medicines that work without side effects against fleas and insect bites, scratching, motion sickness, and ear and eye problems. They also provide hypoallergenic vitamins and trace minerals specific for the very young, adults, and seniors. Canine and feline digestive enzymes and hypoallergenic PURE shampoos are available as well. Dr. Goodpet Laboratories, Inc., Inglewood, CA (800) 222–9932.

Natural Wormer. Solid Gold Homeopet Wormer is a safe product that helps your pets resume their normal activities by ridding their bodies of digestive worms. It consists of natural herbs that remove the physical environment that the worm needs to survive. It contains no chemicals or poisons, so is safe for your pet. Also available are Solid Gold natural dog and cat food and nutritional supplements. Dubl-K-Pet, PO Box 1871, Mishawaka, IN 46546; (800) 382–5573.

Pain Relief for Hip Dysplasia or Arthritis. Glyco-Flex (for dogs) and Nu-Cat (for cats) provide Perna Canaliculus, a safe and natural approach for relieving your pet's discomfort due to hip dysplasia or arthritis. Your pet will gain a greater range of motion, increase in exercise tolerance, and overall improvement in attitude. There are no side effects associated with these products, which are sold through your veterinarian. Vetri-Science Laboratories, 20 New England Drive, Essex Junction, VT 05453.

Pet Food

All-Natural Bird Food. Created in cooperation with (and the official bird food of) the National Wildlife Federation, Wings is the highest quality bird food available for both caged and wild birds. Wings uses only the best seeds while incorporating amino acids, antioxidants, enzymes, vitamins and minerals. Wings contains no artificial ingredients and no fillers like oats, rice, milo (sorghum), buckwheat, "grain products" and other undesirable fillers found in many bird food mixes. Wings is sold in health food, pet, and eco stores and other retail outlets across North America. Natural World Interactions, Inc., PO Box 2250, Halesite, NY 11743–0687; (800) WINGS–67, or (516) 922–5987.

PetGuard's Natural Pet Food. PetGuard is a healthy alternative to commercial pet foods that contains no fillers, preservatives, or animal byproducts. It comes in both canned and dry varieties for dogs and cats. PetGuard also produces vegetarian canned food, Mr. Barky's vegetarian dog biscuits, natural food supplements, and pet care products. PetGuard, Inc., PO Box 728, Orange Park, FL 32067–0728; (800) 874–3221.

Solid Gold's Natural Pet Food. Premium pet food Solid Gold uses amaranth, millet, and barley instead of the allergenic grains of soybeans, wheat, and corn. Also included are healthy canola and flaxseed oils in place of animal and poultry fat which contribute to heart disease and cancer. Solid Gold Hund-N-Flocken dry dog food, a top seller in Germany, was introduced into the U.S. in 1974. This formula is for all dogs, but especially for the dog with allergies or digestive upsets. Cat food and horse products are also available. For a nearby dealer, contact Solid Gold Health Products for Pets, 1483 N. Cuyamaca, El Cajon, CA 92020; (800) DOG–HUND; E-mail: Dane@electriciti.com.

Wholesome Food for Dogs and Cats. PHD (Perfect Health Diet), a complete, balanced full-feed, is a wholesome, meat based diet. PHD has no artificial colorings, flavorings, or preservatives. It does not contain common allergens such as wheat, fish, soy, dairy, and animal byproducts, and our canine formulas are now corn free. PHD has been formulated and endorsed by animal nutritionists, vets, trainers, and alternative practitioners. Ingredients include chelated minerals, kelp, garlic, yeast, barley, oats, lactobacillus, acidophilus, special digestive aids and antioxidants. PHD Products, Inc., PO Box 8313, White Plains, NY 10602; (800) PHD–1502.

Pet Treats

Healthy Cookies. Big Paws pantry offers pet cookies without chemicals, preservatives, artificial colors, or flavors. They hand cut and bake all-natural Companion Cookies from top quality ingredients including garlic, parsley, alfalfa, and oregano. They are available in a wide variety of sizes and shapes and include seven different formulas, three of which are hypoallergenic. Big Paws Pantry, PO Box 727, Duvall, WA 98019; (800) 291–6380.

Holistic Venison Pet Treats. Teddy's holistic venison dog treats are free of all hormones, antibiotic additives, and chemical preservatives. They are made from quality cuts of venison, not inferior byproducts, and come from free range New Zealand animals. Venison bar treats are hickory smoked and individually vacuum packed in 2-ounce portions. Hickory smoked venison bones, in two sizes, also come individually wrapped. Uncle Buck's Venison, Inc., 110 Western Avenue, Henniker, NH 03242; (800) 220–2644.

Supplements, Herbs, and Plant Extracts

Barley Grass Supplement. "Barley Dog" is a powdered barley grass supplement with garlic, nutritional yeast, nineteen amino acids, chlorophyll, proteins, vitamins, trace minerals, and antioxidants. It restores your pet's pH balance, improves digestion, promotes healthy coat, and eliminates bad breath. A portion of sales are donated to Best Friends Animal Sanctuary—the nation's largest "no kill" shelter. Green Foods Corp., 318 North Graves Avenue, Oxnard, CA 93030; (800) 222–3374.

Dr. Halliday's High Endurance and Health Products. A superb energy supplement that includes electrolyte trace minerals, silica, biotin, etc. Easy to assimilate for dogs, cats, ferrets, horses and birds. For complete product catalog: NUTRANIMAL, 7974 Parkside Ct., Jenison, MI 49428. Toll free (888) NUTRITION. (Part of the proceeds goes to Save the Black Rhino Association.)

Enzymatic Food Supplement. The absorption of essential nutrients and fatty acids from pet food is sometimes difficult, making it necessary to add enzymes to the pet's diet. Prozyme consists of lipases, amylases, proteases, and cellulases, and is beneficial to dogs, cats, birds, rabbits, horses, and so on. It is all-natural and scientifically tested to provide maximum absorption of the nutrients needed by your animal. Prozyme Products, 6600 North Lincoln Avenue, Lincolnwood, IL 60645; (800) 522–5537.

Essential Fatty Acid Supplements. This formula replenishes essential fatty acids destroyed by temperature necessary to cook and process food. Animal Essentials contain lecithin, sea bed trace minerals, spirulina plus marine lipids and comes in a liquid oil form. Absolute Nutrition Supplement contains herbs, high protein mineral chelates, vitamins, amino acids, spirulina, and lecithin in a base of stabilized flax seed. If used as directed, these supplements will enhance your pet's immune system. Merritt Naturals, PO Box 532, Rumson, NJ 07760; (888) 463–7748; Website: http://www.merrittnaturals.

Garlic Extract. Kyolic is an odorless, aged garlic product. Its unique aging process changes the harsh compounds and enhances the benefits found in raw garlic, such as its antiviral properties useful in relieving arthritic pain. Other valuable nutrients are found in Kyo-Green, a blend of organically grown young barley and wheatgrasses, Bulgarian chlorella, and kelp. Wakunaga of America Co., Ltd., 23561 Madero, Mission Viejo, CA 92691; (800) 825–7888.

Herbal Supplements for Dogs and Cats. Liquid herbal supplements for both dogs and cats are available from Nature's Answers. These supplements meet the normal needs for natural vitamins, minerals, and trace elements. They contain cell salts, bee pollen, carrots, rice bran, and a multitude of herbs. Also available is Odor Out, which goes to the source of pet malodor (urine) and turns it to nitrogen, oxygen, and water through a molecular change, killing bacteria and preventing flea eggs from hatching. Nature's Answers, 363 Carroll Close, Tarrytown, NY 10591; (800) 395–7134.

Human-Grade Herbal Formulas. These herbal remedies are rich in naturally occurring enzymes that promote a more holistic action on the body. KIDNI FLOW, KIDNI BIOTIC, and KIDNI KARE are effective against urinary incontinence and infections, and help with proper urine production and elimination. LYMPHACARE acts as a blood and lymph cleanser. VIRAL CLEANSE is an antiviral that targets cellular immunity and liver functions, and ADRENAL

SUPREME supports the adrenal system. Holistic Animal Care, 7334 East Broadway, Tucson, AZ 85710; (800) 497–5665.

Liquid Minerals in Electrolyte Solution. PetLyte is a blend of trace minerals in a base of distilled water. Trace minerals in crystalloid form are the key to continuing good health, shiny, healthy fur, good calcium absorption, and a healthy disposition. PetLyte puts the life force back in food and water to fortify the body's defense against chemical additives. Naturopathic Research Labs, Inc., PO Box 7594, North Port, FL 34278; (800) 326–5772.

Natural Herbal Remedies for Dogs. The best remedies often are nature's own, which is the concept behind the first line of liquid herbal formulas for dogs. Tasha's Herbs for Dogs come in concentrated drops that are alcohol-free, palatable, and include flower essences; also available are Adult and Senior Support; The Traveler; Willow Bark Formula; Easy Does It; and Skin and Hair Support. Coyote Springs Co., Box 1175, Jackson, WY 83001; (800) 315–0142.

Nature's Green Food. Bright and Healthy Spirulina is a natural green food that builds strong immune systems and, because of its chlorophyll content, can act as a natural antiseptic and rejuvenator. It contains concentrated amino acids, antioxidants, and more, to satisfy your pet's requirement for live enzyme-producing foods. Earthrise Animal Feeds, PO Box 818, Petaluma, CA 94953; (800) 995–0681.

Nature's Own Folkloric Remedy. Equilite and JBR Equine products are formulated for dogs and cats who are subject to the same bacteria, viruses, or fungi that people are. These products contain a combination of herbs, vitamins, and minerals that enhance overall health. GarliC contains garlic, good against fleas and ticks; astragalus, an immune system strengthener; schlsandra, good for coughs and wheezing; vitamin C; and zinc. Canine Balance assists in digestion, assimilation, and detoxification, and Canine Flex helps dogs with mobility problems, such as pain and stiffness. Equilite and JBR Equine Products, 20 Prospect Avenue, Ardsley, NY 10502; (914) 693–2553.

Necessary Whole Food Supplements. Natural, whole food supplements are necessary for proper nutritional balance. Pines wheatgrass powders or tablets are rich in vitamins, minerals, antioxidants, and enzymes. This product nutritionally resembles a dark green leafy vegetable, but is much more concentrated. It should be a necessary part of your pet's daily diet. Pines International, PO Box 1107, Lawrence, KS 66044; (800) 697–4637.

Nutritional Supplements for Dogs. Nutritional supplementation is needed to strengthen your dog's system. SOURCE PLUS! was designed to fortify your dog against increasing environmental stresses. Its all-natural ingredients include dehydrated seaweed meals, nutritional yeast cultures, and garlic powder. When included in your dog's daily diet, you can expect improvements in allergies, skin and coat condition, and overall health. SOURCE Inc., 101 Fowler Road, North Branford, CT 06471; (800) 232–2365.

Omega-3 Without Fish Oil. Essential fatty acids (Omega-3 and Omega-6) are the building blocks of cell membranes and will help balance and normalize the body. Since they are processed out of most of our foods, we must use supplements. Fortified Flax provides these essential fatty acids from the oil in flaxseed. It is nature's richest source of Omega-3 and this ground whole flaxseed also contains all essential amino acids, high fiber, complex carbohydrates, vitamins, and minerals. Omega-Life, Inc., PO Box 208, Brookfield, WI 53008–0208; (800) EAT–FLAX (328–3529).

Pet Vitamins. If your companion animals' health is compromised by food rich in fats, additives, and preservatives, they definitely need clearing, detoxification, and support. HomeoVetiX formulations have been developed by a pharmacist for natural pet care. They have been "human tested" since 1979 and intensify the innate healing energy of the animal. They are used for allergy and stress control, as well as clearing, detoxification, and nutritional support. Homeo VetiX, 3427 Exchange Avenue, Naples, FL 33942; (800) 964–7177.

Raw Enzymes and Vitamins in a Gravy Mix. NUPRO provides relief for pets with allergies, hot spots, arthritis, poor appetite, anemia, scratching, and itching. This liver-flavored gravy-forming mix includes bee pollen, flaxseed, borage seed, lecithin, garlic, acidophilus, nutritional yeast, and kelp. It contains no ash, sugar, fillers, preservatives, or byproducts, and is highly recommended by many pet owners. Nutri Pet Research, Inc., 8 West Main Street, Farmingdale, NJ 07727; (800) 360–3300.

Super Blue Green Algae. This green food supplies all the essential raw dietary nutrients that are lost in the processing of most animal foods. It is a wild food in a raw, synergistic, organic form providing vital dietary elements necessary for your pet's health. An economical way to get proper nutrition for your animal. Independent Distributors Sharon Trump and Dr. Philip Haselden, 14055 Bicky Road, Orlando, FL 32824; (800) 808–7242.

Therapeutic Yucca Plant. Used for centuries, the yucca plant is an excellent anti-inflammatory and has been proven to be a safe substitute for steroid-based medications. Yucca Intensive liquid is easy to feed to birds, rabbits, ferrets, cats, dogs, farm animals, and horses. It can reduce pain and soft tissue inflammation, eliminate digestive problems, reduce allergic itch, promote tissue healing, and reduce scarring. Holistic Animal Care, 3150 North Lodge Road, Tucson, AZ 85715; (800) 497–5665.

Traditional Flower Remedies. The calming essence and non-addictive effectiveness of flower remedies is well documented. These creams and liquids relieve emotional stress and imbalances, and can act as excellent first-aid products. Five Flower Remedies were discovered by a British physician and have been used worldwide for over sixty years. Bayside Quality Products, 315 Franklin Ave., 2nd Floor, Franklin Square, NY 11010; (888) 724–5489.

Whole Food Pet Supplements. Grown for both human and animal consumption, this unique, broad scope whole food supplement, Pet Total-Lyte, uses a European slow extraction "cracked cell" yeast-culture process. The exceptionally high 70-percent protein factor is further enhanced for absorption by the addition of electrolytesótrace minerals necessary for protein utilization. Electrolytes also provide the catalyst for the body's production of necessary enzymes. Naturopathic Research Labs, Inc., PO Box 7594, North Port, FL 34287; (800) 326–5772.

Miscellaneous

A Little Bit of Everything. Chemical-free living is what every pet hopes their owner will give them. The free Whiskers mail order catalog and store offers a multitude of natural and holistic products from food to frisbees, halters to homeopathy, and everything in between. They are dedicated to providing you with safe, nontoxic alternatives to the products you may currently be using. Whiskers, 235 East 9th Street, New York, NY 10003; (800) 944–7537 or (212) 979–2532.

All-Natural Wheat Kitty Litter. Wheat Scoop is a litter made from 100 percent whole wheat. Active enzymes in the wheat neutralize and destroy enzymes in cat urine, which prevents the ammonia odor. It is dust free and contains no harmful silica, quartz dust, or absorbing clays; it is also flushable and biodegradable. Pet Care Systems, 717 North Clinton, Grand Ledge, MI 48837; (800)–794–3287.

Bau-Biologie and Ecology Courses. The objective of the International Institute for Bau-Biologie and Ecology is to make people aware of the environmental factors in living and work places that have adverse effects on their health, and tell them what to do to overcome these problems. Throughout the United States, they provide correspondence courses, classes, workshops, and seminars leading to certification as a Bau-Biologie Home Inspector, and also offer "healthy house" products. IBE, Box 387, Clearwater, FL 34615; (813) 461–4371.

Carbon-Based Countertop Water Filter. The Aqua Belle carbon-based, countertop water purifier attaches to your faucet and provides protection from lead, chlorine, certain bacteria, and sediment. It is a practical, inexpensive way to protect your pet from ill health due to water contamination. Its replaceable filters last for two years. Aqua Belle Mfg. Co., P.O. Box 496, Highland Park, IL 60035; (708) 432–8979.

Do-It-Yourself Testing Kits for Lead. Test your painted surfaces, dishes, toys, and so on for lead paint with LeadCheck Swabs, and test your water for lead down to 15 ppb (EPA regulation) with LeadCheck Aqua. These self-test kits give you results immediately, as there is nothing to mail away. A toll-free telephone help line can advise you of stores nearby that carry these test kits and can give you advice on your test results. HybriVet Systems, Inc. PO Box 1210, Framingham, MA 01701; (800) 262–5323.

Full-Spectrum Lighting. This type of lighting is the closest lighting to natural sunlight. It provides pets with a natural bright light and heat source that closely mimics the spectrum of natural sunlight. The extra long life Lumichrome bulb emits beneficial ultraviolet rays. This type of lighting is essential to preventing depression in both kennels and homes during the winter. M. Pencar Associates, 137-75 Geranium Avenue, Flushing, NY 11355; (800) 788–5781.

Nontoxic Paints and Sealers. It is necessary to protect yourself and your pets from harmful chemical fumes when you paint or refinish wood. Nontoxic Crystal Aire Sealers and Crystal Shield Paints are water soluble and block out formaldehyde, molds, and other toxic emissions. Allergy Alternatives, 440 Godfrey Drive, Windsor, CA 95492; (800) 838–1514.

Radiant Heat Panels. Enerjoy solid-state radiant electric heating panels are allergy-free and can act as supplemental heating to kennels and pet cages. Designed for whole-house usage, these units operate at 50 percent of the cost of normal electric heat. They are easily installed by an electrician and operate efficiently in well-insulated homes. SSHC, Inc., PO Box 769, Old Saybrook, CT 06475; (203) 388–3848.

Bibliography

A Dish Owner's Guide to Potential Lead Hazards. Oakland, CA: The Environmental Defense Fund.

A Guide to Indoor Air Quality. Washington, D.C.: U.S. Environmental Protection Agency, U.S. Consumer Product Safety Commission, 1988.

A Homebuyer's Guide To Environmental Hazards. Washington, DC: U.S. Environmental Protection Agency.

Ackerman, Lowell, D.V.M. "Enzyme Therapy in Veterinary Practice." *Advances in Nutrition,* Vol. 1, No. 3 (1993).

Amdt, Linda. "The Reintroduction of Whole Living Foods." *Natural Pet Magazine* (March/April 1995): 11.

Anderson, Nina, and Albert Benoist. *Your Health and Your House.* New Canaan, CT: Keats Publishing, 1995.

Anderson, Nina, Alicia McWatters, and Howard Peiper, Dr. *Super Nutrition for Animals (Birds Too!).* East Canaan, CT: Safe Goods Publishing, 1997.

Aontine, W.J., and T. Uno. "Acute Aspirin Toxicity in a Cat." *Veterinary Medical Small Animal Clinical Journal* 64 (1969): 680.

Atkins, Clarke E., D.V.M., and Roger K. Johnson, D.V.M. "Clinical Toxicities of Cats." *Veterinary Clinics of North America,* Vol. 5, No. 4.

Balch, James F., M.D., and Phyllis Balch. *Prescription for Nutritional Healing.* Garden City Park, NY: Avery Publishing Group, 1997.

Beasley, Val R., D.V.M., Ph.D. "Toxicology of Selected Pesticides, Drugs, and Chemicals." *The Veterinary Clinics of North America,* Small Animal Practice, Vol. 20, No. 2 (March 1990).

Bodanis, David. *The Secret House.* New York: Simon and Schuster, 1986.

"Can Your House Make You Sick?" *Popular Science* (July 1992).

"Carbon Monoxide Poisoning." *Medical Essay, Mayo Clinic Health Letter* (February 1984).

"Carboxyhemoglobin Levels in Patients with Flu-Like Symptoms." *Annals of Emergency Medicine* (July 1987).

Casaida, J.E., D.W. Gammon, and A.H. Glickman. "Mechanisms of Selective Action of Pyrethroid Insecticides." *Annual Review of Pharmacology and Toxicology* 23 (1983): 413–438.

Case, Penny. "Flower Power." *Natural Pet Magazine* (November/December 1994): 10.

Claiborne, Ray C. "Teflon and Parrots." *The New York Times* (February 1995).

Clarke, E.G.C. "Lead Poisoning in Small Animals." *Journal of Small Animal Practice* 14 (1973): 183.

Coppock, R.W., L.E. Lillie, and M.S. Mostrom. "The Toxicology of Detergents, Bleaches, Antiseptics, and Disinfectants in Small Animals." *Veterinary and Human Toxicology* 30 (1988): 463–473.

"Contaminant Alert." *Water Technology* (January 1993).

Cremer, J.E. "The Influence in Mammals of the Pyrethroid Insecticides." *Developmental Toxicology for Environmental Science* 11 (1983): 61–72.

Dadd, Debra Lynn. *Nontoxic, Natural and Earthwise.* New York: Jeremy P. Tarcher, Inc., 1990.

Dadd, Debra Lynn. "Put Your Foot Down to Toxic Carpets." *Earth Star* (February/March 1993).

Dahlke, Julie, D.V.M. "A Pet Owners Guide to Common Small Animal Poisons." *American Veterinary Medical Association* (1997).

Dennis, Clue Tyler, and Luke Miller. *If You Like My Apples: A Simple Guide to Biodynamic Gardening.* Garden City Park, NY: Avery Publishing Group, 1997.

"EPA Says 819 Public Water Systems Pose Lead Risk." *Water Technology* (July 1993).

Ertel, Grace. "The Booming Bug Eat Bug Industry." *In Business* (January/February 1995).

"Getting the Lead Out of Your Water." *Better Homes and Gardens* (May 1992).

Goodman, Jerry. "The Alternatives to Modern Pest Control." *Healthy and Natural Journal*, Vol. 2, No. 1: 36.

Gosselin, R.E., H.C. Hodge, and R.P. Smith. *Clinical Toxicology of Commercial Products.* 5th ed. Baltimore, MD: Williams & Wilkins, 1984.

Greeley, Alexandra. "Getting the Lead Out of Just About Everything." *FDA Consumer* (July/August 1991).

Greer, J.M. "Plant poisoning in cats." *Modern Veterinary Practice* 42 (1961): 62.

Heat Recovery Ventilation for Housing. Washington, DC: U.S. Department of Energy, Appropriate Technology Program, 1984.

Hellmich, Nanci. "Experts urge lead tests for household taps." *USA Today* (January 19, 1993).

Hoffman, Ronald L., M.D. "Chronic Fatigue Syndrome Update." *New Life Magazine* (March/April 1993).

"Home Ecology: Carbon Monoxide, a Silent Hazard." *Home Magazine* (October 1993).

"Household cleaners, pest control." *Housatonic Current* (Spring 1994).

"Is your water safe?" *U.S. News and World Report* (July 29, 1991).

Keough, Carol. *Water Fit to Drink: A Guide to the Hidden Hazards of Drinking Water and What You Can Do to Ensure a Safe, Good-Tasting Supply for the Home.* Emmaus, PA: Rodale Press, 1980.

Krenzelok, E.P. "Liquid automatic dishwashing detergents: A profile of toxicity." *Annals of Emergency Medicine* 18 (1989): 60–63.

Larson, E.J. "Toxicity of low doses of aspirin in the cat." *Journal of the American Veterinary Medical Association* 143 (1963): 837.

"Lead-Based Paint Disclosures Are Now Mandatory." *Good Cents Magazine.*

Lee, J.F., G.E. Block, and D. Simonowitz. "Corrosive injury of the stomach and esophagus by nonphosphate detergents." *American Journal of Surgery* 123 (1972): 652–656.

Levenstein, Mary Kerney. *Everyday Cancer Risks and How to Avoid Them: Effective Ways to Lower Your Odds of Getting Cancer.* Garden City Park, NY: Avery Publishing Group, 1992.

Levy, Juliette de Bairacli. *The Complete Herbal Handbook for Farm and Stable.* 4th ed. Winchester, MA: Faber & Faber, 1991.

Martlew, Gillian, N.D. *Electrolytes, The Spark of Life.* North Port, FL: Nature's Publishing, Ltd., 1994.

Martlew, Gillian, N.D. "Is Your Pet Missing Out?" *Naturopathic Research.* North Port, FL: Nature's Publishing, Ltd., 1994.

Mchattie, Grace. *Your Cat Naturally.* New York: Carroll & Graf Publishers, 1992.

McWatters, Alicia. *A Guide to a Naturally Healhty Bird.* East Canaan, CT: Safe Goods Publishing, 1997.

Meyerowitz, Steve. *Water, Pollution, Purification.* Great Barrington, MA: Sprout House, 1990.

Moffatt, Sebastian. "Backdrafting Woes." *Progressive Builder* (December 1986).

Moisture and Home Energy Conservation. MI: Energy Administration Clearinghouse, Michigan Department of Commerce.

Mowrey, Daniel B., Ph.S. *The Scientific Validation of Herbal Medicine: How to Remedy and Prevent Disease with Herbs, Vitamins, Minerals, and Other Nutrients.* New Canaan, CT: Keats Publishing, Inc., 1990.

Newman, Lisa. "Great Clumping Cat Litter . . . Is That Why Kitty Is So Sick?" *Natural Pet Magazine* (March/April 1995): 32–33.

"News from CPSC." Washington, DC: U.S. Consumer Product Safety Commission, 1990.

N,N-diethyl-m-toluamide (DEET); Pesticide registration standard. Washington, D.C.: U.S. Environmental Protection Agency, Office of Pesticide and Toxic Substances, 1980.

Oehme, Frederick W., D.V.M., Ph.D. "Symposium on Clinical Toxicology for the Small Animal Practitioner." *The Veterinary Clinics of North America*, Vol. 5, No. 4 (November 1975).

O'Brien, Robert. "Magic Ions in the Air." *Alpine Air* (1991).

Pedersen, Mike. "POE Systems Reduce VOC Risks." *Water Technology* (August 1994).

Pencar, Mark. "Lighten Up." *Natural Pet Magazine* (July/August 1994).

Pet Care Tips. Ralston Purina Co. (1994).

Petrak, M.L. *Diseases of Cage and Aviary Birds.* Philadelphia: Lea & Febiger, 1969.

Pinckney, Edward, M.D. "Carbon Monoxide Poisoning in the Home." *Vector Consumer Newsletter* (November 8, 1988).

Priester, W.A., and H.M. Hayes. "Lead poisoning in cattle, horses, cats, and dogs as reported by eleven colleges of veterinary medicine in the United States and Canada from July, 1968 through June, 1972." *American Journal of Veterinary Research* 35 (1974): 567.

Ramsey, F.K., et al. "Diagnostic aspects of diseases produced by toxicants in small animals." *Animal Hospital Journal* 3 (1967): 221.

Radeleff, R.D. *Veterinary Toxicology.* Philadelphia: Lea & Febiger, 1964.

Rees, Ann. "Chlorinated Water Linked to Cancer, Study Shows." *The Province* (July 2, 1992).

Renovating Your Home Without Lead Poisoning Your Children. Boston: Conservation Law Foundation.

"Report concludes fluoridated water is safe." *Water Technology* (October 1993).

Reyes, Consuelo. "In our own backyards!" *Cancer Forum,* Vol. 13, No. 5/6.

Riotte, Louise. *Carrots Love Tomatoes.* Charlotte, VT: Garden Way Publishing, 1981.

Ritchason, Jack. *The Little Herb Encyclopedia: The Handbook of Nature's Remedies for a Healthier Life.* 3rd ed. Pleasant Grove, UT: Woodland Publishing, Inc., 1994.

Robb, Maribeth Murphy. "The True Cost of Hard Water." *Kitchens and Bath* (July 1991).

Robbins, P.J., and M.G. Cherniack. "Review of the biodistribution and toxicity of the insect repellent N,N-diethyl-m-toluamide (DEET)." *Journal of Toxicology and Environmental Health* 18 (1986): 503–525.

Rousseaux, C.G., S. Nicholson, and R.A. Smith. "Acute Pine Sol toxicity in a domestic cat." *Veterinary and Human Toxicology* 28 (1986): 316–317.

Safer Cleaning Products. Seattle: Washington Toxics Coalition, 1990.

Scott, H.M. "Lead poisoning in small animals." *Veterinary Record* 75 (1963): 830.

Smith, Charlene. "Green Foods." *Natural Pet Magazine* (May/June 1994): 26.

Smith, Charlene. "How to Treat Common Conditions with Herbs." *Natural Pet Magazine* (May/June 1994): 22.

Smith, Charlene. "Understanding and Choosing Herbal Products." *Natural Pet Magazine* (May/June 1994): 20.

Soyka, Fred. *The Ion Effect: How Air Electricity Rules Your Life and Health.* New York: Bantam Books, 1991.

Sprung, C., and S.T. Kaskin. "Our panel reports." *Modern Veterinary Practices* 51 (1970): 42.

Straight Answers to Burning Questions. Washington, DC: Wood Heating Alliance.

Taylor, Alfred. "Fluoride and Cancer." *Saturday Review* (October 2, 1965).

Temple, A.F. "Bleach, soaps, and detergents." In *Clinical Management of Poison and Drug Overdose,* ed. L.M. Haddad and J.F. Winchester. Philadelphia: W.B. Saunders, 1983.

Tenney, Louise. *Today's Herbal Health: The Essential Guide to Understanding Herbs Used for Medicinal Purposes.* Pleasant Grove, UT: Woodland Publishing, Inc., 1997.

"Treating EPA Regulated Water Contaminants." *Water Technology,* Directory Issue (1995).

Wasserman, B. "Sheep laurel poisoning in the cat—A case report." *Journal of the American Veterinary Medical Association* 135 (1959): 569.

Weissman, Art, and Lisa R. Kruse. "Lead threat may hit 1 in 6." *Asbury Park Press* (August 5, 1993).

What Everyone Should Know About Lead Poisoning. CT: State of Connecticut Department of Health Services.

What Is Antifreeze? Sacramento: California Integrated Waste Management Board.

Wilkinson, G.T. "A review of drug toxicity in the cat." *Journal of Small Animal Practice* 9 (1968): 21.

Wren, R.C., and F.C. Wren. *Potter's New Cyclopaedia of Botanical Drugs and Preparations.* Woodstock, NY: Beekman Publishers, Inc., 1989.

Your Drinking Water—How Good Is It? Cleveland, OH: National Testing Laboratories.

About the Authors

Nina Anderson has a Bachelor of Arts from Monmouth College and is the president of Safe Goods (East Canaan, Connecticut) and the Scientific Alliance for Education. She is a consultant to the building industry, specializing in the promotion of non-toxic construction methods and materials. Ms. Anderson has performed much research in alternative health for over two decades, and has co-authored numerous books on nutrition, successful aging, and the awareness of hazards in the home. In addition, she shares her knowledge through television, radio, and lecture engagements.

Dr. Howard Peiper has a degree in optometry, and now practices in the field of naturopathy. He has studied healthcare issues for over thirty years, and has received national acclaim as a holistic health expert. Among his many achievements, Dr. Peiper co-hosts television's award-winning Partners in Healing, and, with Nina Anderson, has co-authored many books, including works on natural approaches to aging-related problems, Attention Deficit Disorder, and responsible pet care. He is a highly valued lecturer, consultant, and radio personality, as well.

Index

Trouble-shooting for symptoms
and sources of pet poisoning,
3–12
Turpentine, 42
Twitchgrass. *See* Couchgrass.

Vandervort, D. M., 49
Vinegar, 43
Vitamin supplements, 95
Volatile organic compounds
(VOCs), 18–19
Vomiting, 11

Walnut, black, 106
Water
bottled, 83, 88
city, 77–83, 85–88
mineral-deficient, 84, 88
well, 84–85, 89
Water contaminants, 75
in bottled water, 83, 88
in city water, 77–83, 85–88
solutions to, 85–90
in well water, 84–85, 89

Water filtration, 22, 53–54,
85–86, 87
Water hemlock, 58
Wheat grass, 93, 100
Whining, 12
White horehound, 108
Whole-house filtration, 53
Wings, drooping, 6
Wings bird food, 94
Witch hazel, 105
Wormwood, 58
Woundwort, 105

X-ray fluorescence analayzer
(XRF), 52
Xylene, 17, 18

Yeast, nutritional, 71, 93, 100
Your Health and Your House
(Anderson and Benoist),
85
Yucca, 100, 104, 105, 106, 109

Zeolites, 42

Healthy Habits
are easy to come by—
If You Know Where to Look!

To get the latest information on:
- better health • diet & weight loss
- the latest nutritional supplements
- herbal healing & homeopathy and more

COMPLETE AND RETURN THIS CARD RIGHT AWAY!

Where did you purchase this book?

❑ bookstore ❑ health food store ❑ pharmacy
❑ supermarket ❑ other (please specify)_____

Name _____

Street Address _____

City _____ State _____ Zip _____

natural resources

AVERY PUBLISHING GROUP

Trying to eat healthier? Looking to lose weight? Frustrated with bland-tasting fat-free foods?

For more information on how you can create low-fat meals that are packed with taste and nutrition and develop healthy habits that can improve the quality of your life,

COMPLETE AND RETURN THIS CARD!

Where did you purchase this book?

❑ bookstore ❑ health food store ❑ pharmacy
❑ supermarket ❑ other (please specify)_____

Name _____

Street Address _____

City _____ State _____ Zip _____

Headed for Success

Lose Weight
Feel Better
Live Longer

Books for a healthier

RECEIVE YOUR FREE COPY OF HEADED FOR SUCCESS!

1